For Daisyboo and You-Know-Who

Once upon a time there lived a demon in the sky. Any flyer who dared to venture near to his domain was hurled to earth in a fit of demonic fury to lie shattered, crushed and burning on the ground. Through skill and knowledge and the teaching power of time, one being faced and conquered the demon. The demon's name was The Sound Barrier and its domain was Mach 1. From this we learn that demons are only limits and limits are made to be broken.

About this Book

I have divided the journey of this book into two halves. The first deals with the mechanistic attributes and treatments of tinnitus and the second with the reasons *behind the reason* for any bodily discomfort you may experience in your life.

If you prefer, you may dip into this book at will and allow yourself to be led to what you need. Within these pages, as in life, there is no one right way, there is only what is right for you.

1

Introduction

On the 7th of February 2002, I entered the ninth circle of hell. I woke up to something I had never paid any attention to before, Tinnitus. In between crying, praying for restful sleep and total despair I read everything I could on the subject, though no matter how hard I searched, nothing seemed to offer much hope. Doctors dismiss it because they can't see it or quantify it and everyone else seemed clueless. What works for one person doesn't seem to work for another. Beethoven is said to have had it – it is thought that the sound of Tinnitus was all he ever heard in later life since he also suffered from profound deafness. Van Gogh complained of extremely intrusive Tinnitus and cut off his ear. It is just incredibly annoying at best and life-threateningly depressing at worst.

I read that smoking makes it worse. Smoking doesn't change a thing. Ginkgo doesn't help. Stimulants kick-start it. It's in the ear, no, it's in the brain … and time after time people claimed their physicians told them to "Go home and live with it…"

With all these thoughts and theories, despair and rage and frustration, my head was spinning as well as ringing.

I tried to describe it to others. I told them to imagine someone moving into your house and blasting a trumpet on the same high note all day. But wait, there's more. You are tied up on the floor, unable to get to a phone to call the police to have the trumpeter-from-hell thrown out.

No matter which room I went to, I could not get away from the sound. My favourite movies seemed tainted when I tried to watch them. My favourite books were only half-scanned because I had no available attention span. The sound of water running became my sanctuary because it offered me a moment's respite where I could almost remember what silence sounded like.

I have heard there are no atheists in foxholes. I am willing to bet there are no atheists amongst Tinnitus-experiencers, either.

So I asked for help. I prayed, I cried and then I began to study.

One of the most interesting things I learned was from a sound engineer in The Netherlands. He got Tinnitus, suddenly, for no apparent reason, during a meditation class. He nearly went insane before he began his own personal research, ultimately discovering that there is hope. (1)

Another sound engineer in England with Tinnitus, having access to soundproof recording studios, grouped several of his colleagues in one, closed the door and asked them if they heard anything. They claimed they heard nothing, at first, though after a few moments one of them hushed the others and said he heard a high-pitched sound. The others realised they heard it too. I've heard it before in quiet places; everyone has. It's normal.

The British engineer's theory was that some event triggers a sudden awareness of this sound – like a sinus problem, or a blow to the head, or loud noise in a club – and the limbic part of the brain goes "Now that really sucks..." and plays it back extra loudly. The person hearing the brain's feedback (and I know this from my own experience) "Feeds the Beast" with stress, anxiety and fear, making the experience not only distressing, but distressingly continuous.

During the first days of this experience, I was so thankful I had access to the Internet to seek out information and support on Tinnitus. Long ago, people experiencing intrusive levels of Tinnitus must have thought they had been possessed by demons.

The most hopeful thing I learned from a theory standpoint is that it's similar to the times tables in school, like 2x2=4...if you go over it again and again you groove it into your brain and it can take years – or a lifetime – to forget it. In other words, the more attention I gave it, the more it had a chance to groove in.

So my task was to...

Relax. Lighten up. Start doing things I love and stop

worrying. This would give my brain time to forget and regroup those neurons into doing something pleasant. Like remembering Beethoven's Ode to Joy.

One month later, the miracle happened.

I crossed some shining boundary where I wasn't all that bothered. It required lowering my resistance to well-being, and focusing all my concentration on the feeling of relief rather than the frustration the sound produced. For weeks afterwards I never noticed a sound at all.

I recall the day someone said to me, "Well you must have (insert some very long term, which I have since forgotten) and not sound-induced damage to the hair cells like mine."

All I can say in response is that The Night Before The Day After, I had gone to a restaurant for a business meeting in an ultramodern space with stone walls and hard floor and no sound-dampening carpets, curtains or wood. Picture 80-100 people in a concrete bunker augmented by crashing plates from the open kitchen. It was deafening. Everyone had to shout to be heard. I was in there for more than four hours. I woke up the next morning and my life had changed.

One of the main things I learned about the Tinnitus experience is that sometimes when people suffer they want to make delineations of levels, as in, "Well, there's no way you can hurt like I hurt and I am the winner of the hurting contest because…"

People are often afraid that if they try something that works for one person and nothing changes for them, they might end up worse off. It helps them cope with the fear of disappointment in advance. For the longest time, I did the same. Then I learned that the walls I hid behind for protection also cut me off from any possibility of change for the better.

Eighteen months on, I have had several re-occurrences. Each time I go through an abbreviated period of frustration, anger, hopelessness that it "might get worse," but the key term here is abbreviated. I finally figured out that if I can find the sacred quiet once, I can do it again.

Everything changes; the only true absolute of life is change. Anyone can embrace health and well-being as quickly as their opposites. Everything that happens in life is a direct result of the open flow of your desire or resistance to your desire.

Nowadays, if Tinnitus ever enters my consciousness, I make the effort to spend time in aware relaxation. I always wake up the next morning quiet and filled with energy. It is incredibly freeing to discover that you can be in control.

Now I look at my Tinnitus as a smoke alarm for stress – pushing against something you do not desire rather than openly allowing the things you do desire. What you receive depends upon where you place your focus. Stress has made me aware of what I once denied or tried to ignore. When I release resistance and allow the things I desire, my life, my head, becomes peaceful. In this sense, Tinnitus, or any dis-ease of the physical body can be a powerful tool for self-discovery and a profound clue to the seeming mystery that is yourself.

Tinnitus focused me in the Now Moment, and made me aware of what I truly desired more strongly and more insistently than any experience that I can recall. Pain can do that and I think Tinnitus must be a first cousin to pain: relentless, overwhelming, and seemingly never-ending when you are in its midst.

During the early days, I cannot overstate the importance of seeking out and communicating with supportive people who can truly understand what you are going through. Simply discovering you are not alone takes away a huge burden of fear. Beyond a certain point, however, many people find themselves ready to step away from the group for a while, to go further than the concept of comfort in a group experience to a new place. They are ready to discover how to be securely self-reliant in their ability to attain and maintain radiant good health. This book picks up where group comfort leaves off. All that is required is the desire for well-being and a sense of adventure.

Today I bask in my appreciation for my wondrous, self-renewing body. I am basking on the pure white sand next to the calm, quiet ocean of my mind.

Anyone can do what I have done, and more besides.

The only absolute is change and the only firm ground to stand upon is self-love.

2

The Search for Why

Tinnitus is the ultimate symptom of some otherwise undiscovered 'something else.' In many ways, it's like a stuffy nose in that you can tell your doctor about it and he will check down his list... "Got a cold?" he will ask.

"No," you reply.

"Sinus?"

"No."

"Allergies?"

"No."

"Been crying a lot lately?"

"No."

"Eating a lot of wheat?"

"No."

"Been stuffing pencil erasers up there?"

"No."

"Well, I'm sorry, I can't find anything that would be causing your stuffy nose, you'd better go home and just get used to it."

Established medical opinion has left millions of people feeling abandoned, frustrated, and lost in a claustrophobic world of relentless noise. The last true sanctuary, the mind, has been invaded. The impact on quality of life can be devastating.

Strangely enough, this is what I found really liberating, the fact that traditional medicine has hit a wall.

When we go to a doctor we want them to 'Fix it.' Just fix it. I'll spend any amount of money I can if you just fix it. Perhaps someone has to come up with something first that no one else can just fix. Maybe we are pioneers, self-explorers in the true last frontier. Or perhaps I have become a romantic philosopher and can offer you nothing you really want to hear right now. I only feel in my breath and bones that if I can do this, if I can find the quiet for longer and longer periods, you can, too.

What is Tinnitus?

Seemingly relentless sound in the ears and head; buzzing, popping, hissing, roaring, clicking, ringing, and whining are the most common descriptions. The first days are spent vacillating between expecting it to stop at any time and the ever-increasing fear that won't. Concentration and relaxation are the first things to go, beginning a vicious cycle of fatigue compounded by stress, leaving the sufferer even less able to either cope or recover. Social interaction is abruptly curtailed – verbal communication with others is just too much effort over the roar – resulting in feelings of profound isolation. Normal leisure activities like reading, watching television or listening to music are invaded by the ever-present noise. Earplugs can be essential in preventing further sound-induced damage to the ear, but can cause the perceived symptoms to worsen since they block ambient noise and isolate the sound of Tinnitus in your head, making it more noticeable.

It can feel as though the privacy of your mind has been breached. There seems to be no safe place to go, nowhere to run, and less and less hope for change.

The two most important things you can do in the early days are to make an appointment with an Ear, Nose and Throat (ENT) physician and not panic. It could be something as simple as a build-up of earwax or a sinus infection. Really. If, however, the doctor finds no mechanistic cause for the Tinnitus and sends you on your way to deal with it as best you can, You are not alone...

An estimated 45 million people in the US, UK and Europe have some sort of noticeable Tinnitus and at least half that number find that it profoundly affects their daily lives.

In some 10% of cases, the Tinnitus diminishes on its own several weeks after onset with no formal treatment. You could be one of those people. Things can always change for the better just as quickly and easily as not.

One of the fascinating things about Tinnitus is that both the medical community and Tinnitus-experiencers themselves are divided in their opinions regarding where precisely the sound either originates or is perceived. One group says it is caused by trauma to the ear itself, the other is convinced it is either generated or reflected by the auditory, limbic and/or amygdalic regions of the brain.

Tinnitus is usually classified as either objective or subjective. Objective Tinnitus is the rarer of the two and consists of head noises audible to other people in addition to the sufferer. The sound can be caused by vascular anomalies, repetitive muscle contractions or inner ear structural defects and are generally external to the auditory system. An examiner can hear the sound heard by the sufferer by using a stethoscope. TMJ (Temporomandibular joint disease, described in Chapter 3), openings of the Eustachian tubes, or repetitive muscle contractions may also contribute. Pulsatile Tinnitus can be caused by the flow of the carotid artery or the continuous hum of normal venous outflow through the jugular vein and is experienced exactly as named, a pulsing sound sensation. It could be a sign of increased intracranial pressure with additional neurologic abnormalities. The sounds may arise from a turbulent flow through compressed venous structures at the base of the brain.

Subjective Tinnitus may occur anywhere in the brain and/or auditory system and is much less understood, with the causes being many and open to debate. The subjective form is not audible to others. Any area between the ear canal and the brain may be involved.

In any case, every person's experience is unique. The field is wide open to new discoveries. Most of those discoveries are made by people who are living with Tinnitus every day. As in when a person suffers from pain, the experience of Tinnitus is entirely individual and subjective. If you care to consider it this way, there is great freedom in this. For possibly the first time in your life you are in a place to explore exactly what works and does not work for you, what brings you relief and what makes you stronger. You stand to gain valuable skills that will carry you through any experience you may encounter in the adventure of your life. All it takes is self-belief and the desire for change.

What causes Tinnitus?

This is the great question concerning both the medical establishment and individual sufferers.

This section explores the mechanistic approach favoured by current research and seems the best place to begin this journey of self-discovery.

The number one cause of Tinnitus cited by both medical professionals and Tinnitus-experiencers alike, is either exposure to sudden loud noises or progressive hearing loss due to age. It can be a sudden shock from an explosion or blast or sustained extreme exposure from the sound of clubs, concerts, traffic, alarms, drilling, noisy gatherings or, simply, the passage of time and the warranty on your ears reaching the 100,000 mile marker.

The first effect of extreme sound-induced damage is an unusual feeling of fullness or pressure in the ear, similar to being under water. A high-pitched whine or drone usually accompanies the sensation. The full feeling usually subsides, though the ringing tone stays, and in some cases, increases.

Hearing is a series of events in which the mechanism of the ear converts sound waves into electrical signals that are interpreted by the brain as distinct sounds. The three delicate parts of the ear, outer, inner and middle, act in sequence to translate and communicate these signals. A dysfunction in any single part not only affects the final nerve impulse, but the way in which that impulse is interpreted by the brain.

There are three tiny bones in the middle of the ear called the ossicles. They are named the malleus, the incus and the stapes, or by the names usually taught in school, the hammer, the anvil and the stirrup. Acting with the eardrum, they amplify the vibrations, transmitting them to the fluid that fills the snail-shaped cochlea. This fluid moves the top portion of hair cells lining the cochlea, initiating the changes that lead to the production of nerve impulses. These impulses are then interpreted by the brain as sound. Different sounds move the hair cells different ways, allowing the brain to interpret them as distinct.

Sound is measured in units called decibels. Normal conversation is around 60 decibels, the humming of a refrigerator (unless it's my annoyingly loud fridge) is 40 decibels and city traffic can clock in at 80-120 decibels.

Most scientists maintain that sounds of less than 80 decibels are unlikely to exacerbate hearing loss, though it is commonly believed amongst Tinnitus sufferers that there are 'weak' and 'strong' ears, weak ears being more vulnerable to damage.

When damage occurs through noise exposure, and a recovery is experienced within 16 to 48 hours, the period of loss is called a temporary threshold shift. It is believed that a succession of these shifts can ultimately result in permanent hearing loss and/or Tinnitus. Repeated exposure to noise from loud concerts, industrial production or gunfire, anything at a decibel level that causes some immediate discomfort, is cited as a contributing factor.

Recent research shows that hair cells are capable of rebuilding their structure from top to bottom over 48 hours, thus accounting for the temporary threshold shift. When the damage is so severe that it overwhelms the self-repair mechanism, permanent hearing loss occurs.

While all this is happening in the inner ear, what is going on in the brain? Welcome to the "Centrally Based" theory of Tinnitus.

According to this theory, the damaged ear is often the trigger of Tinnitus, the sound not originating in the ear itself, but rather in the way the brain interprets the different (or lessened) signal from the cochlea.

The damaged ear can cause the brain to act as the source of the sound when the brain responds to the altered input from the ear by altering its own activity. The suggestion is that Tinnitus-related brain hyperactivity, once triggered, becomes an independent phenomenon.

The brain, either in an attempt to 'fill in the gaps' from progressive hearing loss or replaying a pattern imposed by sudden, explosive noise, continues with its hyperactivity. It does this because it has seemingly permanently 'rewired' itself in response to the ear damage. This is why severing the entire auditory nerve, which leads from the ear to the brain, often fails to cure Tinnitus. In some cases, the now completely deaf patient is still left with persistent ringing and no ability to mask the sound with ambient noise. This is a grim possibility to consider. Similarly, laser treatments or a cochlea transplant could be no more effective than cutting the auditory nerve, because they would not address the possible source of the perceived sound – the brain itself.

Studies using positron emission topography to chart brain activity have recently confirmed something that researchers have long suspected: in certain people, Tinnitus activates both the auditory and limbic (emotional) centres of the brain. The experience of Tinnitus can raise your blood pressure by inducing anxiety. Sounds trigger emotions, which is why a person can hear a piece of music on the radio and hardly even notice it, while the next selection may bring them to tears. It's all just different sounds, though the emotional response can be very different depending on the exact frequency or combinations of frequencies.

In people who have either habituated or never had a problem with Tinnitus, the sound is like elevator or ambient music – they don't really notice it at all.

In certain horror films, a stringed instrument is often employed to play a sustained high note to heighten suspense. Tinnitus experiencers perceiving a similar sound in their heads may translate this into a sense of dread or anxiety, possibly a trained response by their body to past stimuli. The anxious feelings may then contribute to a greater level of stress, further contributing to the volume or duration of the perceived Tinnitus.

According to the Centrally Based theory, Tinnitus continues, unless one somehow causes re-patterning, or cortical reorganisation, in the affected areas of the brain, thus undoing the effects of the trauma. This re-patterning is most commonly addressed through Tinnitus Retraining Therapy (TRT).

Peripheral (ear-based) Tinnitus is still a possibility. A signal is sent to the brain from damaged ear cells and is then interpreted by the brain as Tinnitus, though the centrally based theory is where current research is headed.

In a 1998 study by Dr Alan Lockwood and Dr Richard Salvi at the University of Buffalo, brain activation was observed corresponding specifically to Tinnitus. They found that when Tinnitus was momentarily increased in one ear due to jaw movements, altered activity was only seen on one side of the brain. While normal sound introduced through one ear would activate both sides of the auditory cortex, Tinnitus appears to activate only one side. This indicates that the Tinnitus signal is fundamentally different from peripheral noise sources, and Lockwood and Salvi concluded that it must be centrally based.

It seems that some people deeply dislike the thought of their brains being 'rewired' and thus tend to gravitate towards the theory of hair cell damage as the source. Conversely, others are frightened of the seeming permanence of hair cell damage and turn with hope to the possibility of re-patterning the brain's perception of sound.

Both scenarios have validity at this point in medical research. Everyone has some hair cell damage and everyone probably has some sort of cortical re-patterning; in terms of both peripheral and central interpretations, it's most likely not a matter of either/or, but more a question of where you believe you are that determines how Tinnitus affects you.

At a certain level, the brain is re-patterned every moment – uncomfortable experiences can be re-interpreted if given the right stimuli. It is also important to realise that your individual experience of Tinnitus at any particular moment does not signify either permanency or increase of the symptoms.

The latest research in peripheral causes seems to be converging around the Dorsal Cochlear Nucleus Disinhibition hypothesis (DCND-H), which maintains that damage to the cochlea leads to reduced neural input for the brain's auditory system. The dorsal cochlear nucleus (DCN), is the first processing station in the central auditory system, contributing significantly to sound processing. Reduced neural input to the DCN results in its becoming disinhibited; put simply, it continues working spontaneously, even when there's no signal for it to process. Disinhibition of this organ is also observed following non-auditory problems involving TMJ disorders and whiplash. The neurotransmitter substances that normally inhibit certain neural activities show reduced action. This absence of inhibition allows increased spontaneous activity of the affected regions of the auditory pathway. Having been sent to the auditory cortex via another crucial organ, the inferior colliculus, this hyperactivity in the DCN is interpreted as Tinnitus.

This may lead to the identification of a final common pathway for the vast majority of Tinnitus cases. This theory focuses on particular organs and locations, and should ultimately include specific neurotransmitter substances as well.

Standing fast against this theory is the supposition that if the process described above is initiated by any and all damage to the cochlea, Tinnitus would accompany hearing loss far more consistently than it does.

It's a mystery. It's a mystery compounded by the fact that a person could have very subtle damage to the mechanism of the ear which has no conscious impact on the capacity for hearing, but which is nonetheless significant for the brain because it slightly alters neural activity. A particular person suddenly perceives an annoying sound, while the next person with a similar level of damage is unaffected.

The correlation between Tinnitus and hearing loss may be due to a specific type of damage, or possibly there is some specific brain chemistry in certain individuals, predisposing them to Tinnitus in response to peripheral triggers.

This can lead us back to the earlier point that Tinnitus is the ultimate symptom for some as-yet-undiscovered 'something else,' and that each person's experience is based on factors completely unique to them and their subjective experience.

I would now like to proceed from the mundane to the possibly super-scary reasons for Tinnitus causes and triggers.

3

Trigger isn't Just a Horse

The Big Four:
Sodium, Sugar, Caffeine, Chocolate

Anything that raises your metabolic rate seems to cause Tinnitus volume to increase, at least in a large majority of experiencers. Caffeine is a stimulant that has a significant influence on cochleovestibular function and has repeatedly shown to be accompanied by increased anxiety. Any increase in anxiety can be read by the body as an increase in stress, aggravating symptoms of fatigue and feeding the vicious cycle of sleeplessness and worry inherent in the early stages of Tinnitus. Elimination of caffeine from the diet can be essential to break the pattern of fatigue and is especially important for the successful treatment with secondary endolymphatic hydrops and for vertigo in those persons with Ménière's disease.

Quinine

The story of quinine and its effects on conquering malarial regions of the planet makes fascinating reading in its own right. Without the antimalarial drugs quinine and mefloquine, the political shape of the world might have been very different from what we see today.

Tinnitus has been noted as a side effect of quinine application in many cases. In addition to Tinnitus, other side effects listed against these drugs include headache, nausea, dizziness, loss of balance, sleep disorders, anxiety, and depression – any of which could aggravate Tinnitus, or contribute to its onset.

A 1991 study gave low doses of quinine to 38 children in

Guinea Bissau to treat Plasmodium falciparum (the parasite that lives and breeds in the stomach of the female mosquito, A.gambiae). Six children reported adverse reactions, mainly mild Tinnitus which disappeared after termination of treatment. A 1995 study of 102 patients with severe malaria noted that the most common adverse effect in those treated with quinine was Tinnitus.

Quinine is also present in minute quantities in tonic water. Many people claim even this amount can trigger their Tinnitus and consciously avoid any drinks containing tonic water.

Red Wine

Some people find it makes it worse, some people swear it helps them cope. If you drink to excess, the stress on your body from the hangover can make the sound of Tinnitus seem louder. Use your best judgement and drink responsibly.

Salicylates

Plants produce salicylates as a way of defending themselves from soil bacteria. Salicylates can be both natural and synthetic (made in laboratories).

Aspirin (acetylsalicylic acid), is taken orally to relieve pain, fever, and inflammation. It is cited by sufferers as the most common cause of Tinnitus in comparison to other non-prescription medications. Some salicylates are applied to the skin in the form of creams, ointments, sprays, or other topical formulations to relieve pain and stiffness in muscles, joints, and ligaments, though the vote is still out on whether it can be absorbed into the body in amounts likely to create a problem. Of further concern are the salicylates in topical creams and ointments for the treatment of common warts and verrucas.

Choline salicylate is used as a gel to treat teething problems in infants, and crosses the line in topical/oral application methods. Nowadays, most parents prefer to play it safe and give their infants a teething ring instead of topical gels for gum irritation.

Foods high in salicylates include berries, grapes and many spices. In the case of grapes, they can fluctuate depending on whether they have been processed. Raw grapes aren't as high in salicylates as raisins and sultanas. Most of the salicylates are in the skin, so peeling the fruit will reduce the amount ingested dramatically. Other foods high in salicylates are apricots, oranges, plums, pineapple, rock melon, all jams, jellies, marmalade and all fruit juices, courgette (zucchini), gherkins, olives, radishes and tomatoes, as well as tomato-based foods such as catsup and baked beans.

Symptoms of mild chronic poisoning (salicylism) include headache, dizziness, Tinnitus, and difficulty in hearing. Excessive or prolonged use of topical preparations containing salicylates can be absorbed into the body in amounts that can cause or aggravate Tinnitus.

Ototoxic Drugs

Certain chemotherapy agents and antibiotics are suspected contributors to inner ear damage and dysfunction. Never be reluctant to question your physician about any medication or treatment you are not completely confident in or comfortable with. Remember, *you hired them to care for you.* You are not just another item on their assembly line. You should always get your time and money's worth in care and concern for your individual situation. Insist on spending enough time with them to get complete and satisfactory answers to your questions and if you feel you are receiving anything less than the finest care, fire them and find another physician.

Non-prescription medications can produce Tinnitus as a side effect as well, without damaging the inner ear. Effects, which can depend on the dosage of the medication, can be temporary or permanent. Once again, before taking any medication, make sure that your prescribing physician is aware of your Tinnitus, and discuss alternative medications that may be available.

The book *Tinnitus: Diagnosis/Treatment* (Lea & Febiger, 1991,

ISBN 0-8121-1121-4) states that ototoxic symptoms may arise days or even weeks after the termination of aminoglycoside antibiotics. Some of the aminoglycosides are Netilmycin and Erythromycin, Colistimethate, Doxycycline and Minocycline.

The following is a list of drugs that have demonstrated Tinnitus side effects as indicated in the 1995 *Physicians Desk Reference* and distributed by the American Tinnitus Association:

Accutane, Acromycin, Actifed with Codiene Cough Syrup, Adalat CC, Alferon, Altace, Amicar, Anatranil, Anaprox and Anaprox DS, Anestacon [among most common], Ansaid, Aralen Hydrochloride, Arithritis Strength BC Powder, Asacol, Ascriptin A/D, Ascriptin, Asendin, Asperin, Atretol, Atrofen, Atrohist Plus, Azactam, Azo Gantanol, Azo Gantrisin, Azulfidine [rare]

BC Powder, Bactrim DS, Bactrim I.V., Bactrim, Blocadren, Buprenex, BuSpar,

Cama, Capastat Sulfate, Carbocaine, Cardene [rare], Cardioquin, Cardizem, Cardura, Cartrol, Cataflam, Childrens Advil, Cibalith-S, Cinobac, Cipro, Claritin, Clinoril, Cognex, Corgard, Corzide, Cuprimine, Cytotec, Dalgan, Dapsone, Daypro, Deconamine, Demadex, Depen Titratable], Desferal Vials, Desyrel & Desyrel Dividose, Diamox, Dilacor XR, Dipentum, Diprivan, Disalcid, Dolobid, Duranest, Dyphenhydramine [Nytol, Benydrl, etc], Dyclone, Dasprin,

Easprin, Ecotrin, Edecrin, Effexor, Elavil, Eldepryl, Emcyt, Emla cream, Empirin with Codiene, Endep, Engerix-B, Equagesic, Esgic-plus, Eskalith, Ethmozine, Etrafon,

Fansidar, Feidene, Fioricat with Codeine, Flexeril, Floxin, Foscavir, Fungijzone,

Ganite, Gantanol, Gantrisin, Garamycin, Glauctabs,

HIVID, Halcion, Hyperstat, Hytrin,

Ibuprofen, Ilosone,Imdur, Indocin, Intron,

Kerione,

Lariam [among most frequent], Lasix, Legatrin, Lncocin, Lioresal, Lithane, Lithium Carbonate, Lithobid, Lithonate, Lodine, Lopressor Ampuis, Lopressor, DCT Lopressor, Loreico, Lotensin HCT, Ludiomil,

MZM [among most frequent], Magnevist, Marinol (Dronabinol), Marcaine Hydrochloride, Marcaine Spinal, Maxaquin, Mazicon, Meclomen, Methergine [rare], Methotrexate, Mexitil, Midamor, Minipress, Minizide, Mintezol, Moduretic, Mono-Cesac, Monopril, Motrin, Mustargen, Mykrox,

Nalfon, Naprosyn, Nebcin, Neptazane, Nescaine, Netromycin, Neurontin, Nicorette, Nipent, Nipride, Noroxin, Norpramin, Norvasc,

Omnipaque, Omniscan, Ornade, Orthoclone OKT3, Orudis, Oruvail,

P-A-C Analgesic, PBZ, Pamelor, Parnate, Paxil, Pedia-Profen, Pediazole, Penetrex, Pepcid, Pepto-Bismol, Periactin, Permax, Phenergan, Phrenilin, Piroxicam, Plaquenil, Platinol, Plendil, Pontocaine Hydrochloride, Prilosec, Primaxin, Prinvil, Prinzide, Procardia, ProSam, Proventil, Prozac [infrequent],

Questran, Quinaglute, Quinamm, Quinidex, Q-vel Muscle Relaxant Pain Reliever,

Recombivax HB, Relafen [3-9%],Rheumatrex Methotrexate, Rifater, Romazicon, Ru-Tuss, Rythmol,

Salflex, Sandimmune, Sedapap, Sensorcaine, Septra, Sinequan, Soma Compound, Sporanox, Stadol, Streptomycin Sulfate, Sulfadiazine, Surmontil,

Talacen [rare], Talwin [rare], Tambocor, Tavist and Tavist-D, Tegretol, Temaril, Thera-Besic, Thiosulfil Forte, Ticlid, Timolide, Timoptic, Tobramycin, Tofranil, Tolectin, Tonocard, Toprol XL, Toradol, Torecan, Trexan, Triaminic, Triavil, Trilisate, Trinalin Repetabs, Tympagesic Ear Drops,

Ursinus,

Vancocin HCI, Vantin, Vascor, Vaseretic, Vasotec, Vivactil, Voltqaren,

Wellbutrin,

Xanax, Xylocaine [among most common],

Zestril, Zestoretic, Ziac, Zoloft, Zosyn, Zyloprim

Benzodiazapines

In order to help the patient cope with the anxiety

accompanying the onset of Tinnitus, doctors often prescribe a family of drugs known as the benzodiazapines. These can include Lorazapam (Ativan), Klonopin, Xanax, Valium or Restoril.

It is of the utmost importance to slowly taper off any usage of these drugs when stopping or changing medications. Benzo withdrawal can make the Tinnitus seem worse since the drugs directly affect the areas of the brain that cope with anxiety.

Benzodiazapines are a heaven-sent gift to many sufferers since they may allow them the calm, quiet space necessary for the deep inner work that is vital for recovery.

Anything you do that reduces the anxiety associated with Tinnitus is a valuable tool. Choosing a tool that helps you – and this includes prescription medication – is not 'cheating' and it doesn't earn you fewer gold stars for enlightenment.

Sinuses

What are Sinuses?

The sinuses are hollow cavities found in the bones of the head and face. Sinuses start developing right after birth and keep growing for the first 20 or so years of life.

Sinuses lie adjacent to the nasal cavity and are therefore anatomically named the "paranasal" sinuses. Four sets of sinuses lie on each side of the nasal cavity: frontal, ethmoid, maxillary, and sphenoid sinuses. The frontal sinuses occupy the bone over the eyes in the forehead while the maxillary sinuses are under the eyes in the cheekbones. The ethmoid sinuses are actually a collection of sinuses, like a honeycomb, lying between the eyes. The sphenoid sinuses are placed behind the nasal cavity and eyes, near the centre of the head.

The paranasal sinuses are similar to rooms lying off a main hallway, the nasal cavity. Air flows up and down this hallway as we breathe in and out through our noses. A special "wallpaper" lines the nasal "hallway" and each sinus "room." This lining is the mucosa, which swells and thickens with irritation or inflammation. The sinuses are connected to the hallway through very narrow openings, sometimes only one or two millimetres wide. When the "wallpaper" lining these narrow openings swells, it can block the openings and result in a sinus infection.

What is the Purpose of Sinuses?

Sinuses help add moisture to the air you breathe and give depth or tone to your voice. Every day, a quart or more of mucus slides from your sinuses into the back of your nose and down your throat. Naturally, anyplace in your body that is both warm and humid as well as having immediate exposure to elements outside the body can be a breeding ground allowing invading organisms to establish and grow. When the moisture-filled mucus no longer flows because of a cold or sinus infection, the sinuses become blocked and the resulting pressure can create a ringing sensation that can be perceived as centred in the ears and Eustachian tubes.

The simple answer to the question regarding the purpose of sinuses is that no one knows for certain. Many theories have been proposed, all of which may be correct.

By creating air-filled chambers within the skull bones, the sinuses may serve to decrease the weight of the head. They also add resonance to the voice; when they are blocked we sound like we are talking through our noses. The sinuses also form a sort of "crumple zone" that can protect the eyes and brain in case of a severe injury to the face.

The second most commonly prescribed medication, after pain treatments, are the drugs to treat or alleviate the symptoms of hay fever, colds or sinusitis. Unfortunately, many of these medications are cited as causing or aggravating Tinnitus. Exploring alternative treatments such as acupressure, massage, cleansing, herbals and homeopathic medicine have proven to be effective for many people, thus avoiding the risk of creating Tinnitus symptoms or aggravating an existing condition. Any tool is valid if it works for you.

Spinal Pressure

Take your hand and place it on your forehead, press firmly against it, increasing the tension on the back and sides of your neck. If you hear a difference in the sound volume of your Tinnitus you could be storing stress in the upper shoulders and neck.

Nerve compression in this area is a very common response in people who literally shoulder their life burdens and live in expectancy that "the axe will fall" at any moment.

The healthy spine is a marvellously balanced mechanism of discs, nerves and fluid augmented by the muscles, ligaments and tendons of the back, carrying nerve impulses from the brain to every part of the body. It is the main communicative channel between the mind and the molecules of our physical being. Any blockage of this superb communicative system can result in stuck energy, translated as stress and interpreted as pain.

The first and most important place to begin in order to achieve spinal health is to pay attention to your posture. Good posture balances all the systems of the body, all organs are in their proper places and able to function at peak efficiency. When you achieve a constant awareness of your posture, and gently return to the feeling of balance each time you slump into the old habitual crumple, you will no longer be straining the muscles supporting the back and can begin to allow the unimpeded flow of communicative signals between your mind and the cells of your body. You will maximise the vitality of your immune system, sharpen your awareness and improve your general emotional outlook by a factor of, oh, one bazillion...

Good posture really is that important.

Our spine is the main communication superhighway, via the nervous system, between mind and cells, yet if we go through our life and charge through the day with our shoulders up around our ears, bracing ourselves for the next blow, shuddering with relief at having made it through another hellish day and finally collapsing into an exhausted heap before a partial descent into restless sleep, we are short-changing ourselves of the best life has to offer.

Of immediate benefit to Tinnitus experiencers, the awareness of good posture can decrease the volume of the sound simply through tension relief. Relief can also be found in prescribed medications, consciously performed relaxation techniques and/or getting plenty of solid sleep. Tension caused by stress has been shown in most Tinnitus experiencers to be a major contributor to both volume and duration of the sound. Achieving and maintaining proper posture and spinal balance can be one of the most important steps you can make towards achieving and maintaining the sacred silence within.

TMJ

Temporomandibular joint disease – a painful condition affecting the area where the lower jaw connects to the sides of the skull, impairing function and sensation in the face and jaw, which may spread to the ears, neck, and shoulders and exacerbate T volume.

Jut your lower jaw forward as far as you can and hold for several seconds...does the volume increase? You may be holding tension in your Temporomandibular Joint. You have lots of company. An estimated 20 million people in the US, UK and Canada suffer from TMJ and the majority, as high as 90 percent, of TMJ patients are women in their childbearing years.

Medical research has not yet defined all the causes of TMJ. Certain dental or medical procedures, oral habits, injury, and a variety of joint diseases and disorders like arthritis, can precipitate or aggravate TMJ.

The Symptoms of TMJ:

Facial pain; jaw joint pain; often in combination with neck, shoulder, back pain and/or headaches as well as pain when opening or closing the mouth, yawning widely and chewing.

Popping, grating or clicking sounds with movement of the jaw joint

Swelling on the side of the face and/or mouth

A bite that feels uncomfortable.

Limited opening or inability to open the mouth comfortably

Deviation of the jaw to one side or the inability to swallow easily.

Vertigo, visual difficulty or disturbances and diminished hearing are also cited by TMJ sufferers, though many of these symptoms may often indicate a different disease process occurring simultaneously.

The most commonly noted trait shared between back/spinal problems, TMJ and Tinnitus is the presence of tension from the interrupted processing of stress.

Stuck energy, translated as stress and interpreted as pain by a body crying out for better communication with the mind, is a clue that we may desire change, but simultaneously fear that same change in case it could be 'for the worse.' This can keep us forever with one foot on the fuel pedal and the other on the brake, doing nothing, going nowhere, straining our physical vehicle to the breaking point.

Diving

Tinnitus is one of the most prevalent and bothersome of symptoms related to diving. It can be related to temporomandibular joint pressure from clamping down on the mouthpiece, wax build-up in the ear canal with tympanic membrane irritation, barotrauma to the middle and inner ear or decompression illness involving the inner ear. It is most often found in association with vertigo (dizziness) and there is usually some deafness.

If you develop problems with diving-related Tinnitus, go for a full examination by a diving-oriented ear, nose and throat doctor. Check or change your regulator mouthpiece to achieve a proper fit and be aware if you are clamping down on the mouthpiece. You can try clenching your teeth and notice whether or not you hear a high-pitched whine when you do.

If you indulge in nerve stimulants like excessive amounts of coffee (caffeine) and smoking (nicotine), they might be best avoided the day before and for 24 hours after diving.

Pressure-induced damage to the delicate inner ear system can also be a contributing factor. Know your individual safe dive level and do not exceed it.

If the Tinnitus persists or worsens during or after each dive, you might consider giving it up and taking up skydiving instead...with ear protection from the wind noise, of course.

Ménière's Disease

Ménière's disease is usually characterised by four main symptoms: periodic episodes of vertigo or dizziness, fluctuating, progressive, low-frequency hearing loss, Tinnitus and a sensation of "fullness" or pressure in the ear.

Periodic attacks of vertigo can the most disruptive of the symptoms to the patient. It is usually the vertigo which causes the patient to seek medical treatment. Typically, vertigo occurs in the form of a series of episodes over a period of weeks or months, interspersed by periods of remission of variable duration.

The episode can consist of a period of dizziness, unsteadiness or the perception of spinning. The sensation of spinning may produce a beating of the eyes from side to side, nausea, vomiting, sweating and all the symptoms normally associated with extreme motion sickness. The onset of the episode may be preceded by a sensation of fullness or pressure in the ear, increased hearing loss and a sudden Tinnitus 'alert' sound. The onset is frequently sudden, reaching peak intensity within minutes and lasting for an hour or more before subsiding. Unsteadiness may persist for hours afterwards.

The person experiencing vertigo may perceive either that the world is spinning around them or that they themselves are spinning. Vertigo disrupts virtually every aspect of life, since the patient can lose the ability to accomplish most normal tasks, particularly where muscular movement is involved. In addition to the obvious fear of falling, the experiencer can be hampered by the fact that even small head movements often make the spinning sensation worse.

The accompanying nausea, sweating and/or vomiting combine to make the patient subjectively extremely ill. Vertigo can incapacitate the sufferer to the point that they are no longer able to function effectively, leaving them with a feeling of helplessness compounded by illness.

Most people are familiar with mild forms of dizziness from carnival rides, spinning in place, or round dancing. In a healthy individual the effects may last for up to 30 seconds. With Ménière's disease, the same unsteadiness can last for days, confining the person to bed for the duration.

One of the main difficulties of the Ménière's disease experiencer is the dread accompanying the fear of when the vertigo might return. This stress can add yet another layer of suffering on top of the existing situation, exacerbating the torment. A feeling of helplessness characterised by individuals with Ménière's disease is compounded by worry that the 'other shoe will drop' when they least expect it, leading, in some cases, to a self-fulfilling prophecy.

Unable to recover because of the worry, and worrying that they are unable to recover begins a vicious spiral into despair.

This can be a truly desperate place to be, no less intrusive than Tinnitus alone, and just as socially isolating. The interior compass of an individual experiencing Ménière's disease is spinning, seemingly out-of-control, with no true north to key on.

Low Frequency Hearing Loss with Ménière's Disease

The hearing loss associated with Ménière's disease often affects one ear, typically with a loss of sensitivity to low-frequency (bass) sounds. Sounds may be perceived as muffled, distorted, or "tinny." Loud sounds may cause more discomfort than normal, moving into hyperacusis (intolerance of 'normal' sound). This can also fluctuate over time, becoming either less or more noticeable due to fatigue or accompanying illness. Because the hearing may improve and worsen from one day to another, the experiencer's anxiety may increase because of the uncertainty over what to expect next, and the worry about whether it will change for the worse. Also, the degree of hearing loss may become more serious with time, eventually affecting all sound frequencies. Hearing may eventually seem to be completely lost in the affected ear.

One of the most useful things the Ménière's sufferer can do is to drink an adequate amount of pure water. Though it may seem excessive if you are accustomed to drinking coffee, tea or soft drinks, 8-10 8oz glasses of pure water per day will replenish fluid losses caused by the stress of the body attempting re-balance itself. As well as giving the kidneys and related organs the chance to thoroughly cleanse the blood and lymphatic systems, drinking plenty of pure water will ease the stress on the affected aural and central nervous systems. It is also important to anticipate and replace large fluid losses that occur during exercise, illness or when the weather is hot. Pure water is your best friend where the re-balancing physical body is concerned.

If your physician prescribes diuretics as part of your treatment, this is done not to cause you to lose fluids but rather to encourage your kidneys to excrete a constant amount of urine throughout the day, thus helping to minimise big swings in the body's fluid content. You may need to take a potassium supplement along with the diuretic in order to replace potassium lost through increased urination.

Medications may also be given to help control your dizziness, nausea, and vomiting, if those symptoms are a problem for you.

In all cases of prescribed medications, plenty of pure water is essential in both helping the medications do their proper jobs and cleansing the body of accumulated toxins from stress. You can still find the level place within, the sacred silence and eternal balance. Illness is due to resistance and resistance is characterised by stress.

People diagnosed with Ménière's Disease are thought to have endolymphatic hydrops; however, not all people diagnosed with endolymphatic hydrops have Ménière's disease.

Endolymphatic hydrops is a disorder of the vestibular system of the inner ear. It stems from abnormal fluctuations in the fluid which fills the hearing and balance structures of the inner ear.

In a healthy inner ear, the fluid is maintained at a constant volume and contains specific concentrations of sodium, potassium, chloride, and other electrolytes. This fluid bathes the sensory cells of the inner ear and allows them to function normally.

If the inner ear is damaged by disease or injury, the volume and composition of the inner-ear fluid can fluctuate with changes in the body's fluid and electrolyte levels. This fluctuation causes the symptoms of hydrops—pressure or fullness in the ears, Tinnitus, hearing loss, dizziness, and imbalance.

The treatment of hydrops involves stabilising body fluid levels so that secondary fluctuations in the inner ear fluid can be avoided.

The amount and composition of your inner-ear fluid is affected by the salt and sugar concentrations of your blood and other body fluids. Eating a balanced diet in moderate amounts at regular intervals can help ensure that your salt and sugar levels remain fairly stable. You may also need to modify your diet to decrease sodium intake.

Regarding the possible causes of hydrops, they can include a blow to the head, infection, degeneration of the inner ear, allergy, or, rarely, a tumour.

Acoustic Neuroma

Acoustic neuroma is a benign tumour arising from the vestibular nerve. Common symptoms are loss of hearing, Tinnitus and ataxia. An audiogram may show increased pure tone average, increased speech reception threshold and decreased speech discrimination. MRI scans commonly show a densely bright tumour in the internal auditory canal. Treatments include surgery, radiosurgery and sometimes simply observation. For radiosurgery, multiple smaller treatments rather than one large treatment are options.

The most common response to discovery of an acoustic neuroma is rushing into surgery. This is not always the best or most necessary option. The best advice, as always, is to not panic.

Many acoustic neuromas grow very slowly, and some do not grow at all after being diagnosed. Almost all patients can afford to wait 6 months and to find out their acoustic neuroma's rate of growth, though naturally you must discuss this point with your physician.

With the current pace of improvements in research, monitoring and tumour treatment-specific drugs, it's worth taking your time to examine all your options if the tumour is not growing quickly.

Surgical outcome depends more on the experience of your physician than on anything else. It's worth seeking out a specialist who can maximise the odds of a good outcome. Acting out of panic may land more newly diagnosed acoustic neuroma patients in rushed and unsuccessful surgeries than anything else.

Patience with yourself and holding on to the certainty that good health is your birthright has been proven in many cases to be essential for the best possible outcome.

Three Terms You might have come across in Your Personal Research

Misophonia, Phonophobia and Hyperacusis are three aspects of the same condition, a perceived hypersensitivity to all or certain sounds.

Hyperacusis

Hyperacusis is diagnosed when a person complains of everyday sounds being at an unbearably uncomfortable level, even when the same sound, such as normal conversation, is at an acceptable level for everyone else.

Misophonia

A person may not be painfully sensitive to conversational

decibel levels or ambient sounds of nature, like waves crashing on the beach, but claim that particular noises set off a discomfort response, no matter the decibel level. Traffic, electronic activity in media systems, construction noise or loud appliances are the most commonly cited examples.

Phonophobia

If the dread or dislike of certain sounds affects the experiencer to the point of extreme panic at the thought of actually hearing them, and this panic in turn affects their normal day-to-day functioning efficiency, the term phonophobia is applied as a valid psychological categorisation of their condition.

The Fringe Contingent Weighs in

The Schumann Resonance Frequency has been described as the heartbeat of the Earth. Though it can vary among regions, for decades the measurement was 7.8 cycles per second. This was once depended upon to be a constant, though recent reports set the current rate at over 11 cycles, and this rate appears to be increasing every year.

Science acknowledges that the Schumann Resonance is a sensitive indicator of temperature variations and world-wide weather conditions and is believed by many people to go hand-in-hand with the increase in severe storms, floods, and weather of recent years.

Any phenomena affecting the earth to this degree can also have an effect upon the creatures living upon the earth, and the adjustments our bodies may be either making or resisting during this process of change can have profound effects upon our physical systems, including aural or neural processes.

The earth is changing. We choose whether or not to embrace or resist those changes.

Electromagnetic frequency fluctuations and increases can include the widespread use of cellular phones and masts, increasing microwave transmissions and current low frequency wave research.

Most people believe that living near huge electrical pylons can have adverse effects on our health. Added to that, the increased use of cell phones and the corresponding increase in the number of relay masts – often erected in the middle of residential neighbourhoods – contribute to a massive increase of electromagnetic radiation in our environment. Many people and communities are concerned with the possible health effects of this, which are not well understood. In these first years of burgeoning electromagnetic bombardment, the jury is still out on the toll it could be taking on our health.

There are very few places to run and hide on this planet, but it could be recommended that you take a month off, get as far off the grid as you can and assess whether or not you observe a difference in the way your body feels. You might be pleasantly surprised at your recovery, and even consider changing your entire lifestyle to include a more low-tech approach to living.

If this is not an option for you, be aware of the amount of time you spend in the company of electromagnetic fields generated by televisions, computer monitors, sound systems, appliances and heavy wiring in sound studios or editing suites, and pay attention to the way your body responds. Spending time amongst trees, fresh air and moving bodies of water may help considerably, relieving the stress that modern communications, manufacturing and entertainment can exacerbate.

Our bodies, guided by our minds and inspired by our spirits, are marvellously adaptable and capable vehicles for our souls on the journey of life. Throughout human history we have only scratched the surface of discovering the miracles we can accomplish.

4

Tinnitus DIY

So you've seen your doctor, you may have tried what they've suggested, and either nothing seems to change or they offered you very little hope. You have now arrived at a place where it is clear that if anything is going to change, it's up to you.

For the remainder of this book we will explore what you can do, on your own, both inner and outer work.

Recently, technology and advances in traditional medicine have provided an abundance of resources designed to help Tinnitus experiencers in coping with and eventually moving beyond the stress and into freedom and rediscovering the sacred silence within.

Further Resources

Many people with Tinnitus also have hearing loss, and wearing a hearing aid can make it easier for them to hear the sounds they need to hear by making them louder. The theory is that the better you hear other people talking, or the more clearly you hear the music you like, the less you notice your Tinnitus.

Maskers are small electronic devices, worn like hearing aids, which emit sound to make Tinnitus less noticeable. Maskers do not cure Tinnitus, but they can make the perceived Tinnitus sound seem softer. For some people, maskers hide their Tinnitus so well that they barely notice it.

People who are helped by masking the Tinnitus sound report better and more restful sleep. Adequate rest is essential for emotional health during the first few weeks of the Tinnitus experience. Devices which you can put by your bed include a radio tuned to soft static, as well as masking sound generators specifically designed for the use of Tinnitus experiencers. Natural ambient sound CD's are good as well, particularly ones featuring running water or waves on the seashore. Ear pillows, a recent development, work in a similar way, generating white or pink noise when the head is placed on the pillow, and can be particularly helpful if the Tinnitus is perceived primarily on one side of the head or the other.

Speaking of ambient sound, there is a joke amongst T experiencers that they must be the cleanest people in the world because of the near universal feeling of relief obtained by listening to the sound of running water. Hot showers can also be helpful by clearing blocked sinuses that may contribute to the feeling of fullness and the sound of ringing. Anything you can do to contribute to your feeling of relief will be time well spent in first relaxing your body, then retraining your brain to perceive new sounds in place of the Tinnitus noise.

Relaxation Techniques

The second and third sections of this book deal with this in some detail. I cannot overstate the importance of learning to create peace with the present moment. When you have developed the skill of selectively choosing what you feel and knowing the power you can hold when using your brain as the tool it was meant to be, your entire universe becomes a playground. There is so much beauty in your universe. Your only job is to allow it in.

Medicine or Drug Therapy Scientists are currently studying how changes in blood flow in the cochlea affect hair cells. When a person is exposed to loud noise, blood flow in the cochlea drops. However, a drug that is used to treat peripheral vascular disease maintains circulation in the cochlea during exposure to noise. These findings may lead to the development of treatment strategies, thus easing the effects of Tinnitus. If your doctor prescribes medicine to treat your Tinnitus, make sure they tell you whether the medicine has any other side effects.

Tinnitus Retraining Therapy

This treatment uses, amongst other methods, a combination of counseling and masking techniques. Otolaryngologists and audiologists help you learn how to understand and cope with your Tinnitus. They may also recommend maskers to make your Tinnitus less noticeable. The eventual goal is to train your brain to avoid thinking about Tinnitus. An investment of time is required for this treatment to work, but it has proven to be very helpful – most publicly by the actor William Shatner, who recently completed a course in the treatment method pioneered by Dr. Pawel J. Jastreboff, and who claims complete success with the programme.

According to Dr. Jastreboff, habituation begins with attaching a noise generator the size of a hearing aid that makes a low-level sound just below the volume of the individual's Tinnitus. The device is worn eight to 10 hours a day for 18 to 24 months. During that time, according to Jastreboff, the brain undergoes "plastic" changes, reprogramming itself to tune out the sound; in the process, the Tinnitus is "tuned out" as well. If treatment is successful, the patient is no longer aware of the sound of Tinnitus.

Counseling

People with Tinnitus may become anxious, depressed or suicidal. Talking with a counselor or fellow experiencers in Tinnitus support groups may be helpful. With access to the Internet, there are many wonderful options for finding and utilising information and support.

Alternative Treatments

Massage

Stress has been found to make tinnitus worse, so anything you can do to relieve your stress is definitely good. This includes massage, though as in any relationship where quality communication is important, it may take several attempts to find a therapist that is skilled at bringing out the best results in both of you, but when it's right, when it's a good match, you will know it. You may then wish to discuss your Tinnitus in depth, asking your therapist to pay particular attention to the back of your neck and upper shoulders, both of which are common places to store tension.

You might also investigate the current practice of including small hot stones placed at key points on the back of your body during the massage. These have the added benefit of targeting specific meridians having to do with the flow of chi (qi). The goal with chi, otherwise known as life force, is unblocking and balancing this flow in order to allow your body to reclaim its naturally healthful state. Besides, those little hot rocks feel really, really good.

For self-massage, pay special attention to your feet. Doing this during a bath is good, because you are relaxed and possibly even listening to running water at the same time.

Take your time with this, notice any especially tender points between your toes or at the ball of your foot and…rub. Not with too much force, but with a sort of tender conviction. A good self-massage session with your feet can show astonishingly immediate results as well as helping you learn what your body specifically requires to maintain balanced health.

Acupuncture

In order to understand how acupuncture works, it is helpful to become familiar with the basics of Chinese philosophy. In order to understand how well it works, you only need to have it performed by a qualified acupuncturist with a good reputation. The philosophies of the Tao, yin and yang, the eight principles, the three treasures and the five elements are all fundamental to traditional Chinese acupuncture and its specific role in helping to maintain good health and a person's well-being. A good acupuncturist will be well versed in these philosophies and strive to communicate their skills through the principles of rebalancing the natural healing tendencies of your body.

Acupuncture is the practice of inserting very fine needles into the skin to stimulate specific anatomic points in the body. Along with the usual method, the practitioner may also use heat, pressure, friction, suction, or impulses of electromagnetic energy to stimulate the points.

In the past forty years, acupuncture has become a well-known, reasonably available treatment in the Western Hemisphere. It is neither scary, invasive or painful when practiced by a qualified acupuncturist and most people report experiencing a feeling of profound relaxation both during and after the procedure.

Acupuncture and acupressure (fingertip pressure applied to the same anatomic points as acupuncture) may help decrease the perceived level of Tinnitus sounds you hear, possibly through relaxation and rebalancing. In traditional Chinese Medicine, Tinnitus is believed to result from a disturbance in the flow of energy to the liver or kidney

Homeopathy

In the Fourth Century, Hippocrates, the father of modern medicine, observed that large amounts of certain natural substances can produce symptoms in healthy people resembling those caused by disease, while smaller doses of these same substances can relieve symptoms of the same illness. Nearly fourteen hundred years later, the German doctor Samuel Hahnemann, studied this concept and proposed the practice he named homeopathy, allowing like to be cured by like. The name homeopathy comes from the Greek word "homios" which means "like" and the word "pathos" meaning "suffering". Homeopathy uses animal, vegetable and mineral preparations to help the body to heal. Millions of people agree with this concept and make the homeopathic approach a vital part of their lives.

The basic theory is that substances that are poisonous in large doses can be very beneficial in small doses. The objective is to prevent the patient from getting the illnesses again. Homeopathic practitioners look at each patient's symptoms, lifestyle and emotional state and develop a remedy or treatment plan strictly for him or her. At its most effective, Homeopathy encourages the powers of healing inherent in individuals via the immune system and the more the practitioner knows about the patient, the more successful the treatment.

Homeopathy has a lot in common with our present understanding of immunisations. To prevent us from catching small pox, a vaccine is prepared using a crippled form of the virus that causes the disease. The understanding is that by introducing this small amount of the virus into the body, it will stimulate the body's defences so that we will be immunised when and if the smallpox virus tries to enter. Homeopathy practitioners believe that when we introduce a nearly infinitesimally small amount of material into the body via homeopathic preparations, our body will also unleash enough defences to prevent disease without adverse reaction to the actual substance itself.

There are, however, significant differences between the concepts of immunisation and homeopathy. Vaccines are not rendered more potent when they are diluted. In vaccine and antibiotic treatments, there is a minimum dosage that needs to be given before the medication becomes effective. Homeopathic remedies, on the other hand, are diluted to such an extent that there can be no possible side effects from even the most toxic substances. Taken in this ultra diluted form, Homeopathic remedies have no side effects and are perfectly safe, non-toxic and non-addictive, though the body, in its inherent desire for balanced health, still responds with favourable, and often astounding, results to the diluted form of the homeopathic treatment.

The most popular recommended treatments for Tinnitus include:

Calcarea carbonica: Tinnitus may be experienced alone or with vertigo; Possible hearing problems and pulsing sensations in the ears; usually chilly, easily fatigued, crave sweets, feel overwhelmed when unwell.

Carbo vegetabilis: Ringing in the ears during flu, vertigo or nausea; may feel worse in the evening; feel cold and faint, though crave fresh and moving air.

Chininum sulphuricum: Buzzing, ringing, and roaring sounds loud enough to impair the person's hearing. A tendency toward chills and vertigo, during which the Tinnitus is worse.

Cinchona officinalis: Nervous with sensitivity to noise; accompanying Tinnitus; fluids have been lost through vomiting, diarrhoea or heavy sweating.

Cimicifuga: Very sensitive to noise; accompanying Tinnitus; Pain and muscle tension in the neck and back; full of nervous energy and talkative, but depressed or fearful when not feeling well.

Coffea cruda: Excitable, nervous; accompanying Tinnitus with extremely sensitive hearing; buzzing feeling in the back of the head. Often accompanied by insomnia from mental overstimulation.

Graphites: Tinnitus with associated deafness. Hissing and clicking sounds are often heard in the ears. A tendency toward constipation, poor concentration, and cracking skin eruptions.

Kali carbonicum: Tinnitus with ringing or roaring, accompanied by itching in the ears and vertigo; feeling anxiety in the area of the stomach.

Kali phosphorica: every hour for buzzing and/or humming, or ringing after nervous exhaustion.

Kali. Sulph every 2 hours during the evening to relieve nighttime Tinnitus.

Lycopodium: Humming and roaring in the ears; impairment of hearing; sounds seem to echo; ear infections with discharge; chronic digestive problems or urinary tract complaints.

Mag phos for whizzing and ringing and where hearing is limited.

Nat. Mur. Use 3X or 6X potency, taken several times a day for humming or singing sounds.

Natrum salicylicum: Ringing in the ears is like a low, dull hum; vertigo may be involved. Useful when Tinnitus and tiredness occur after influenza or along with Ménière's disease.

Salicylicum acidum: Tinnitus with very loud roaring or ringing sounds accompanied by deafness or vertigo. Flu and Ménière's disease are other indications. This may also be helpful if Tinnitus has been caused by too much aspirin.

Herbal Medicine

Okay, let's get this part out of the way.

If you're reading this book, then you obviously have good sense. You presumably don't want to become a Darwin Award winner and you like feeling good and taking responsibility for your own health and well-being. That said, here are a list of precautions I feel compelled to add regarding Herbal Medicine.

Never take essential oils internally. Avoid contact with eyes and private parts and other sensitive areas when using essential oils or herbs. During pregnancy, check with a traditional medical doctor before using any essential oil or herb. If you suffer from high blood pressure, epilepsy, are currently taking prescription medication or a course of antibiotics or are habitually accident-prone with a tendency for self-destruction, check with a doctor before using essential oils or herbs. Never use undiluted essential oils on the skin. Never use essential oils or herbs on or in infants and small children without professional guidance. Should you suffer an adverse reaction to any essential oil or herb, stop using it immediately and contact a medical practitioner or poison control centre.

Feel better? I do. Thank you for indulging me.

An herb is a plant or plant part that is prized for its medicinal, aromatic or savoury qualities. Herbal medicine is the oldest form of healthcare known. Herbs have been used by all cultures throughout history. As time went on, each culture developed their discoveries of the medicinal powers of plants, promoting a huge diversity of knowledge regarding effects upon the body.

Beginning in the 18th century, much of this knowledge was built upon by refining the active properties of the plant and eventually synthesising and patenting the processes necessary to transform the raw plant into uniformly standardised amounts.

Herbal medicine is a major component in most indigenous peoples' traditional medicine and a common element in Ayurvedic, homeopathic, naturopathic, traditional oriental, and Native American Indian medicine. Substances derived from medicinal plants remain the basis for a large proportion of the commercial medications used today for the treatment of heart disease, high blood pressure, pain, asthma, and other health challenges.

One of the problems with these refined substances is that each plant is a carefully balanced system of chemicals that work alongside the active ingredient to augment its effects. One example of this is with cocaine. In its original form, coca leaves, it is a harmless stimulant used by the indigenous peoples of South America for centuries. In its refined form, with uncontrolled use, it is recognised as a potentially highly addictive health hazard.

Conversely, one of the problems with using the raw form of the plant is that levels of active ingredients can vary tremendously according to where and how the plant was harvested and its drying method and processing before ingestion. Without self-education, you could find yourself completely dependent upon the quality of the herbalist who prepares and dispenses your herbal treatment.

Interest has been growing in recent years from reported success stories in the use of herbs to treat illness, discomfort or distress. One example, St. John's Wort, is widely used in the treatment of mild depression without the need for medications such as Prozac. In trial after trial, St. John's Wort does not show the side effects of Prozac and could therefore be a more desirable alternative.

The following list of Herbal Remedies has been tried, discussed and found to be useful in many cases. If you buy your herbal remedies in capsule form, you may wish to stay with the same brand each time you buy, since this will go quite a ways towards ensuring uniform dosages. Most companies find a good source, establish a method of preparation and afterwards, stick with it. Also note any warnings, instructions and use-by dates on the bottle and adhere to these rigorously.

Ginkgo Biloba

Ginkgo has been found, in some studies, to be useful in minimising the distress of Tinnitus although other studies have failed to find the same results. In Europe, trials have confirmed the use of standardised ginkgo extract for a wide variety of conditions associated with ageing, including Tinnitus, vertigo, memory loss and poor circulation, so follow your best instincts and decide whether or not to give it a try. If it eases some other distress, it could create a domino reaction of healing of which Tinnitus is a symptom.

On the other hand, Ginkgo has been shown to be an extremely potent blood thinner. It is not recommended for use by people with any type of bleeding disorder, and/or presurgical patients. To compound Ginkgo with other medications that may be physician-prescribed, such as Coumadin or Plavix could lead to disastrous results. Ginkgo is a medication to be very careful with. If Ginkgo is a choice you have decided to embrace, plan to invest some time in taking it as it is known to work slowly.

Sesame

Sesame seeds have been used by Chinese herbalists and in Indian Ayurvedic treatments for Tinnitus, blurred vision and dizziness. Since it very affordable and can be added to food it is a cost-effective and, barring allergy, safe addition to the herbal list.

Black Cohosh

There is some anecdotal evidence that black cohosh in decoction form is useful in alleviating Tinnitus. Many herbalists recommend that black cohosh be used in combination with ginkgo for best results.

Goldenseal

Do not use goldenseal if you are pregnant. Herbalists recommend the use of goldenseal and black cohosh in combination, one to one.

Lesser Periwinkle (Vinca minor)

The lesser periwinkle contains a compound known as vincamine. Extracts containing vincamine have been used in Germany to help decrease Tinnitus and Ménière's disease symptoms. There are some severe side effects noted with overdosage of this herb. In animal tests, changes in blood counts were observed. It is recommended that if you take this herb, you should do so under the advice and care of a professional.

Spinach (Spinacia oleracea)

Ingesting spinach and other foods containing zinc may be beneficial in the treatment of Tinnitus. Good sources of zinc include spinach (the best), papaya, collards, Brussels sprouts, cucumbers, string beans, endive, cowpeas, prunes and asparagus and sesame seeds.

Sunflower Seeds

Traditional Chinese medicine calls for eating sunflower seeds and drinking a tea brewed from their hulls for Tinnitus. If you do brew tea from the hulls, strive to make sure they are from an organic source to avoid ingestion of pesticides.

Fenugreek Seed Tea

Drinking a cup of fenugreek seed tea three times a day is reported to abolish disturbing ear noises.

Passion flower

Passion flower extract is known to regulate neurotransmitters and circulation, both shown to be crucial factors in some cases of Tinnitus.

Horsetail

Supplementation with vegetal silica, an aqueous extract from horsetail, has been found to decrease Tinnitus.

Chinese Herbs

Coptis and Rhubarb Combination (San-huang-hsieh-hsin-tang): Prescribed for Tinnitus due to hypertension.

Important: Herbs to Avoid

Avoid aspirin or aspirin-like herbs — willow bark, meadowsweet and wintergreen. High doses of aspirin (acetylsalicylic acid) may cause ringing in the ears. Other herbs that are suspected to aggravate Tinnitus include cinchona, black haw and uva ursi.

Hypnosis

For people who find it easy to slip into a meditative state, hypnotherapy can be a very effective treatment. The main function of a talented therapist is as a guide, and it is crucial that you feel comfortable enough with them to form a trusting relationship. In the trance state, your therapist should be able to help you to visualise your Tinnitus as easily controllable, perhaps the same as adjusting the volume dial on a radio.

Bach Flower Remedies

Dr. Edward Bach was an avatar of all that is great and holy about being a healer. Feeling dissatisfied with the way doctors were expected to concentrate on diseases and ignore the people who were suffering them, Bach abandoned a lucrative Harley Street practise and followed his heart, which led him ultimately to Oxfordshire, in the English countryside, on a botanical odyssey. Following his keen intuition, he discovered the remedies he wanted, and – this is the crucial difference in his approach to healing – each remedy was aimed at rebalancing a particular mental state or emotion in the patient.

The wonderful thing about these remedies is that they appear to work so well for so many people. In the midst of a

Tinnitus episode characterised by despair, Bach's Rescue Remedy can help bring the balance necessary to approach and embrace true healing. For specific emotional issues discovered on your personal journey, read the descriptions of emotional states addressed by each of the remedies and choose which is right for you.

Ayurveda

According to Ayurveda, there can be no mental health without physical health, and vice versa. Symptoms and diseases that could be seen as thoughts or feelings are just as important as symptoms and diseases of the physical body, if not the same thing in two aspects.

Ayurveda is India's traditional system of medicine. Ayurveda is a Sanskrit word that literally translated means "science of life," developed and practiced for more than 5000 years through observations, experiments and discussions. For several thousand years the teachings were passed on orally, but in the fifth to sixth century BC detailed texts were written in Sanskrit.

Ayurveda emphasises prevention of disease, rejuvenation of our body systems and extension of life span. The profound premise of Ayurveda is that not only can we prevent disease, we can also better understand ourselves and the world around us, in balance and harmony with all life and that, with self-love, live unafraid of expressing our true inner nature.

Ayurveda is based on the view that the elements, forces, and principles that comprise all of nature are also a part of our physical and emotional bodies. In Ayurveda, the mind and the body not only influence each other – they are each other.

Together, the mind-body is an integral part of the universal consciousness, the aware ocean of energy that gives rise to the physical world we perceive.

The philosophy and practice of Ayurveda link us to every aspect of ourselves, and, in turn, every aspect of the universe. In Ayurveda, the division between self and other is consciously imposed, and illness can result from the attempt to force those divisions into place and hold them there, unchanging, out of a fear of the unknown.

According to Ayurvedic tradition, Tinnitus is a vata disorder. To alleviate this aggravation of vata in the nervous system, a tea prepared from equal amounts of comfrey, cinnamon, and chamomile is recommended. Steep up to 1 teaspoon of this mixture per cup, and drink 2 or 3 times a day.

Home Remedies

Increase circulation to the ear area by massaging or applying a hot compress on the neck before going to bed. Dip a small towel into hot water, wring out, place on neck and place a dry towel over it.

Stimulate overall circulation with alternating hot and cold foot baths every evening.

Place a small cotton pouch filled with 3 tbsp. each of hot roasted millet seeds and salt on one ear. Leave on for ten minutes.

Gently rubbing the mastoid bone behind your ear with warm sesame oil may be helpful. Try it twice a day, morning and evening, for a week.

Place three or four drops of castor oil in each ear before bedtime and insert a cotton plug.

5

Tinnitus Past and Present

Jonathan Swift, author of Gulliver's Travels, revealed in a passage in his journal that he had the symptoms of Ménière's disease, a condition that benefits from a low-salt diet. He stated that good food needed no added salt except where it was necessary for preserving meat in long voyages. He knew he benefited greatly from avoiding it. From youth, he suffered from severe attacks of giddiness, described well enough to permit a confident diagnosis of Ménière's syndrome.

In December 1888, the French newspaper *Le Monde*, in a story about Vincent Van Gogh, described his infamous ear-cutting and subsequent giving of that ear to a woman named Rachel. Much debated, many describe this action as madness, but closer inspection of his letters indicate that he suffered from Ménière's syndrome, a build-up of fluid in the inner ear that causes vertigo, nausea, and ringing in the ears. Before antibiotics, patients sometimes pierced their eardrums with ice picks in an attempt to ease the pressure and stop the noise.

Health Magazine of Nov./Dec. 1993 reported that the painter Francisco de Goya complained bitterly of an incessant roar in his head after becoming deaf in 1793. He channelled his torment into his art, creating portraits and studies of angry characters holding their hands over their ears.

Czech composer Bedrich Smetana described his Tinnitus, or ringing in the ears, as a 'shrill whistle of a first inversion chord of A-flat in the highest register of the piccolo' as he translated his agony to the world. His lead violin plays a piercing high E through much of the finale in his first string quartet in E minor.

The 19th century British physician, Joseph Toynbee, credited with being the father of otology (the study of the anatomy and diseases of the ear), was found dead after inhaling chloroform in an attempt to relieve his Tinnitus.

Beethoven, Martin Luther and Francis Bacon all suffered from Tinnitus. In Beethoven's case he was entirely deaf; the only sound he heard near the end of his life was the incessant roar in his head. The composer Robert Schumann also had Tinnitus while Charles Darwin kept daily records of its amplitude and frequency. Thomas Edison was plagued with his Tinnitus, also noting it in daily journal entries.

The list of present day personalities who have Tinnitus is a long one, and seems dominated by people in the music industry. I have gathered the names mentioned here from Newspaper, Magazine and Internet sources. I have never met or interviewed anyone listed below.

According to the various print, broadcast and Internet media I researched, Tinnitus experiencers include Neil Young, who mentions Tinnitus as the main reason for his move from electrically-amplified music to acoustic. Barbra Streisand also has Tinnitus, as well as Engelbert Humperdinck, Sting, Brian Wilson of the Beach Boys, Jeff Beck, Eric Clapton and Lemmy Kilminster of Motorhead who is quoted as saying, "We just like it loud, you know?"

In an interview, Eric Johnson stated that he'd, "...run two Marshall stacks onstage and crank the monitors. I started using Fender Deluxe Reverb amps and 50-watt Marshalls around '97, after I started having some problems with Tinnitus. It was my own doing—being irresponsible and thinking I was invincible...though it has been better lately. Take care and wear plugs. Don't think it can't happen to you. When I had a speaker re-coned at the been-here-for-years re-coning shop in Austin, the owner said, 'I've re-coned speakers for every guitarist in Austin for years and as far as I know there aren't any rock 'n roll lead guitarists here who don't have Tinnitus to some degree or another. Many have it so bad they have trouble sleeping.'" (2)

Other musicians with Tinnitus include Dave Pirner, Bob Mould, Liberty Divito, guitarist James Hetfild (who swears by his Sonic II ear plugs) and drummer Lars Ulrich. Tim Bogert, bassist, is quoted as saying that he has '…Tinnitus, big time…'

Kevin Shields, guitarist and singer says that his damage occurred listening to mixes in headphones at very loud levels without giving his ears time to recover.

John Densmore of the Doors has been a long-time sufferer, as well as Ted Nugent, George Harrison, Graham Cole, and George Martin, who retired from music due to hearing loss.

Bono writes about his Tinnitus, as seemingly noted in select lyrics for his band, U2.

Phil Collins has had to cut back on live performances '…thanks to the buzzing in his ears…'

Ozzy Osbourne, Cher and Huey Lewis are on record as having suffered the effects of Tinnitus both currently and in the past.

Charlie Haden, jazz bassist, talks about suffering from Tinnitus, which he attributes to having played an especially tumultuous version of free jazz with the tenor saxophonist Archie Shepp and the trombonist Roswell Rudd in the late 1960s, as well as hyperacusis, both conditions leading him to position himself behind Plexiglas baffles when playing with a drummer. (3)

Haden also reports that over the years he has learned to adjust his life to accept his ear problems as part of his being and to tell himself that he's been this way since he was born. He claims this helps him reduce the stress and frustration of the condition. He goes on to note that he wears earplugs that cut out 32 dBs and wishes fellow sufferers good luck and advises them to keep a positive outlook.

Blinda Butcher, bassist and singer, states that she "…had a punctured ear drum which fortunately they were able to put right, but for a while I couldn't hear out of one ear and it was very depressing. On stage we all wear hearing protection and encourage anyone who sees us to do the same." (4)

Michael   Tomlinson,   musician/singer-songwriter, temporarily lost 90% of his hearing for a few weeks after an ear infection, but still has Tinnitus in one ear.

Non-musicians suffer as well. A short, yet wide-ranging list includes Ronald Reagan, Former First Lady Rosalyn Carter, David Letterman, and actors Sylvester Stallone, Neve Campbell, Burt Reynolds and Jerry Stiller. The late Alan Shepard, first American astronaut in space, also had Tinnitus. Actors Tony Randall and Richard Thomas, as well as musician and actor Steve Martin has Tinnitus. Newsreader Peter Jennings and writer Clive Barker both have it.

Tinnitus experiencers compass the entire range of ages, mediums and geographical locations. Tinnitus is a truly universal experience. The scale may seem skewed towards sound-induced hearing damage, but many people in the music industry never suffer at all while others, never knowingly exposed to loud sounds, can suffer as well.

Whatever discomfort or dis-ease you may be experiencing, whether or not it has either a traceable cause or no apparent explanation, all illnesses have the same thing in common: They are signs of imbalance, discrepancy or resistance between the mind and the body. It is truly as simple as that. Not always easy, just simple.

The moment your desire for change is greater than your fear of change, you can accomplish miracles.

Sources

1   Rob van Heelsbergen
    http://homepages.onsnet.nu/~robvh/tinnitusE.htm
2   Adam Levy, Guitar Player Magazine, September 2001
3   Charlie Haden, Bass; Francis Davis, The Atlantic Monthly, August 2000
4   The Grateful Deaf; Jay Babcock, MOJO Magazine, December 2000. Mirrored at www.jaybabcock.com

And Here is Where it Begins to Get Fun...

6

Mach 1

Your brain is a tool. Everything you think you know is processed by the brain as experience and either embraced or rejected by you, via your mind, as beliefs. That is all reality ever is and ever will be: what you believe it is.

Life is a Self-Guided Tour

This life you are living is a self-guided tour. Religion, philosophy, science and art offer side excursions of their own on this tour, and you can subscribe to any of these you like, at any time you choose. You are also free to make up your own tour, with its unique itinerary of experiences. No one ever stops you from doing exactly that except yourself.

You may be considering enjoying aspects of my tour as I present them in the form of this book. And why is this my tour? Simply because this book is full of my beliefs – that is, my beliefs as they exist at the time I am writing this. When these beliefs no longer serve my best desires, well, maybe I'll write another book. Or maybe I'll just keep quiet and have a wonderful time anyway. It's my choice to write or not and your choice to read or not. Freedom's great that way.

For the present, some of the ideas in this book may resonate with you and the experience you would like to have, some you may furiously reject. That is your right as well. Everything you think and feel has always been your right and your choice, and always will be.

Everything you ever experience is always your choice.

You may choose to travel with the excursion tour offered by a religion. If this enhances your life then it is a good thing. If someday you are ever interested in creating your own path it would be good to remember that all religions are a series of events characterised first by the birth of a good idea. This idea gradually develops into dogma architected by other humans and finally ends up carved into the rock of Rules-You-Must-Adhere-To-Or-Else by still more humans. The original good idea came from a human, just like you. They had a really Good Idea about how the world could work and shared it with other people. Those people then took it and ran with it and eventually developed it into the Rules Carved In Rock.

These good ideas end up as rigid rules primarily because people in general aren't convinced of the value of their own ideas. They believe they are floundering in an ocean of uncertainty and it can seem much safer to cling to the same rock others are grasping with such apparent fervour, the presumed Rock of Absolute Truth.

Absolutes make people feel safe. Absolutes can't be argued with or challenged. Absolutes seem to be a secure place to hide.

Absolute Truth also seems to be different everywhere you go. Looking closer, Absolute Truth seems to be different for every person you ever meet. Wars are fought over which Absolute Truth is the correct one. Absolute Truth is debated in courts all over the world every day. Many religious texts claim to hold the Absolute Truth, and the debate over which text is correct has been the number one cause of violent death on this planet.

Why are there so many different religions and philosophies, styles of art and architecture and music? Why are there so many seemingly contradictory scientific theories? Why are there so many customs and cultures and beliefs? And what does all this have to do with your Tinnitus? Because life, without choice, is no life at all and illness is a choice as much as health. All these different creations – or none of them – are choices to be selected or passed over by you on the Self-Guided Tour of your life.

Whether you heal or not, whether you are rich or not, whether or not you have a joyous relationship with another person, everything you experience in your life is a direct result of whether you embrace your worthiness to make the choices that will bring you the most joy while simultaneously allowing others to do the same.

When a person observes that a belief which serves another's happiness may not necessarily satisfy them, or what may have served in the past is no longer what they now desire, the first true spark of change is born. What trips people up, time and again, is fearing the very change they desperately desire.

Humans have a hunger to create more and better and different experiences all the time. It's really the entire point of being alive. The difficulty comes because people, by and large, are terrified to do it alone, to be the first to try, to stand out from the crowd, to march to the sound of their own drummer and shake their booty to their own brass band. They are afraid of making – first four notes of Beethoven's Ninth here, please — A Wrong Decision.

Despite all the warning labels, home and car insurance, new laws preventing this or that, eating lots of fibre or belonging to the right religion, country club or political party you will never make the world safe enough if you spend your life expecting to be hurt.

What is Driving You
(and why aren't you doing the driving instead?)

What spurs many people on when they first realise their lives have got to change is feeling stuck in a rut and frustrated with everything. You don't have to let it get to that point. The simple fact that you desire a different experience should be enough. You don't have to let the beliefs that you don't deserve any better than what you already have make you angry enough to change. Anger never accomplished anything but drawing more of the same.

You might desire more money or better health or a loving relationship and no matter what you try, nothing seems to get any better. Often, before you have floated very far away, you turn right around and paddle back to the rock you were clinging to before, living out the popular principle that the devil you know is better than the devil you don't. And there you remain.

Many people then use the frustration they feel as an opportunity to beat up on themselves emotionally. Or they use the frustration they are feeling to try and change other people. Or they turn this frustration to physical destruction. The pain of focusing on their own lives and their seeming inability to do anything about that pain is too great to bear. Some people bury themselves in busywork and projects, squashing and denying and distracting themselves from the suffering. The only thing the running and doing and distracting and avoiding can ever do is make you exhausted enough not to care that you are hurting.

The Myth of the Martyr

It doesn't have to be difficult, or painful or exhausting. Pain and fear are habits you've been holding on to. They are beliefs. That life appears painful or fraught with danger is a simple belief, and can therefore be changed.

Determined to change something, anything, about their lives, many people often resort to using force in order to make their desire happen. They force themselves to do their duty. They work and strive and suffer when it's so much simpler to allow your desires to happen. By allowing what you desire to come to you, you remove the burden of having to **make** things happen by forcing them. Simply allowing your desire is not only possible, but infinitely more pleasurable and efficient. It is only your belief that life is hard, success comes with a price, it's lonely at the top, that make them true for you.

Do you know the first person to ever say, "No pain, no gain," to you was someone that wanted you to work towards their agenda?

Still, the idea of suffering gets very big press nowadays. In one of the larger organised religions, martyrdom has been glorified to the point that they give out big prizes for it called "Sainthood." I suppose there is some satisfaction in getting your face on a medal or having a building named in your honour, but the main two problems with sainthood are:

1. You only get it after you're dead, and
2. You have to suffer a lot to qualify, like, bleeding from your palms or getting leprosy or being burned at the stake. Plus, no sex. Lots of no sex. Or at least not ever getting caught having sex.

In the media, the story of The Survivor is a very fashionable theme. Miraculous survival stories abound. Movies are made about survival, chat shows are devoted to discussing the heroics of people who have survived, hundreds of millions of dollars are awarded in courts on the basis of it. Being a survivor has a certain seductiveness about it. It has the scent celebrity, of being taken care of, and just the faintest aroma of being right and justified and admired. And considering all the money awarded in settlements all over the world, it can be lucrative to be a victim. Being a victim and a survivor is one of the modern interpretations of sainthood.

This book is not about being a survivor. It is about being a thriver.

Thrivers don't need to be rescued. They don't need to sue anyone for damages. They don't need a building named after them. Thrivers no longer need the contrast of drama to be filled with joy. Thrivers are ready to let go of the need to be a victim. Thrivers don't need to be acknowledged the winner in a debate or to be seen by the world as being justified. Thrivers aren't motivated by anger. Thrivers aren't driven by a need to fulfil something they think is lacking in either themselves or the world. Thrivers enjoy life for the pure, endless fun of desiring, creating and allowing in the manifestation of their creations. Thrivers know there is no competition with any other person for anything they could ever desire, unless they desire to play it that way for the fun of competition.

Thrivers know there is an endless supply of energy and love

and light, laughter and money, health and abundance available to them at all times without depriving any other being of anything that being desires to experience in their own lives.

Victims see lack because they choose to see lack. Some of you are here reading now because you may have felt that Tinnitus happened to you and now you are the victim of Tinnitus.

I am here to say that as long as you believe that, it will be true for you.

The moment you are willing to let go of that belief, you will begin to allow in the wellbeing that exists all around you, all of the time. That will be the very moment you will begin to rediscover the Sacred Quiet. It truly is all up to you. It has always been your choice. It always will be.

For the present, suffering may be what you choose to do. This is your right. It is always your right to choose what you experience from your self-guided tour.

If you find that it's not working out for you anymore, that suffering is not making you any happier, when you find you are tired of being in pain, you are immediately faced with re-evaluating your beliefs about the nature of reality. Specifically, **your reality,** and the part that fear plays in your reality.

Fear

Desiring change and fearing change at the same time and with the same amount of passion guarantees that nothing either very good or very bad will ever happen to you. For many people this is the comfort zone where they prefer to live their lives. Boredom seems a very small price to pay for what appears to be relative safety and secure predictability.

What other people think, though, and how they choose to live is not your concern. You are your concern. For you, frustrated and in pain, uncertain of what you desire nor how to create it, inhabiting your body can be like sitting in a car and pressing the fuel and the brake pedals at the same time. You aren't going to travel anywhere very efficiently and will ultimately only cause wear and tear on the mechanism. Your body is the vehicle your spirit travels around in here on earth and it is suffering under the strain of this frustration.

When you are ready to believe in the worth of your own desires, you can experience what once seemed to be a sea of uncertainty as an ocean of choice. You can reach the point where making those choices no longer seems fearful. You let go of the rock you've been clinging to and are suddenly free to swim, or float, to step onto an unknown shore or bask on the beach or explore the beckoning land, to build a boat and sail, to do anything you've ever dreamt of doing. Or you could continue to cling to the rock with everyone else who thinks the way you do. As always, that is your choice.

Your life is the only life you can ever change. You are the only person who can decide when the time is right to effect that change. You are the only person who knows what you truly desire.

The trick is focusing on what you do want and not on what you don't.

The obstacle is fear.

What do You Fear Most?

Pain? Uncertainty? Death? Ridicule?

In my own experience and from my own observations, the biggest fear most people ever have might be the realisation that they are alone. We all die alone. We all suffer pain alone; no one can do either for us. Neither can they know exactly what we see with our eyes or hear with our ears or dream when we sleep, no matter how we strive to communicate those things through poetry, painting or music. No one knows exactly what you feel, and how you feel it, but you.

The search for a soulmate often translates into the desire to somehow alleviate that feeling of being utterly alone in the experience of life. That every soulmate you may ever meet ultimately transforms into just another human with their own roster of fears and desires can leave you feeling even more alone than before the relationship and further inclined to seek the sanctuary of cynicism or bitterness.

You are alone. You are alone because you are an individual having an experience called life that is completely unique to you. You are alone because despite the begging, pleading, lying, seducing, dominating or manipulating you may do, you can never really change another human being. You are alone because the only life you can ever have an effect on is your own. You are alone because you are suffering, you've sought help from your doctor and been told there is nothing they can do for you.

Once you have it absolutely clear in your mind that you are alone, you can see how liberating it is to be free of all responsibility over another person's experience. When you face the fear that you are alone, and that it is perfectly okay to be alone – even desirable most of the time – then you will be free to see all the possibilities for creating a joyous life of your own, very personal, design. Only then will you be free to enjoy the company of others without fear of ever being hurt again, free of obligation, guilt or the need to use force or seduction to alter what you perceive as the other person's problems. You will be free to realise that everything you ever experience, including your health, is an endless series of opportunities to create precisely what you most desire. You will begin to add to the sum total of beauty in the world by your radiant health and obvious happiness about just being **you**, every moment of the day. This will become apparent in the way that people begin to respond to you; babies will laugh when you walk into the room, dogs will wag their tails, strangers on the bus will smile. Some will be drawn to you and others who used to irritate you will wander off and find someone closer to their own vibration to hang with. Most fascinatingly of all, you will realise that you effect greater change upon the world and its inhabitants not by fighting or protesting, campaigning, proselytising or preaching, but by simply being happy. Instead of vibrating down to the status quo, you vibrate up to your own capacity for joy and others who are ready to do the same will be drawn to you effortlessly.

This realisation, that you are alone and it's actually a very good thing is the second most positive step you will ever take on your journey. The first most positive being loving yourself exactly as you are in this now moment. When you realise that you are perfect, nothing needs to be forgiven, you are in the perfect place at the perfect time and all is really well, then you will know you have never really been alone at all, you have always had yourself. The walls of resistance you have been holding up for protection will dissolve and you will allow that which you most desire to come to you.

Tinnitus, or any other health problem, is a signpost of imbalance between your mind and your body. It is an urgent message your body is sending you that something needs to be looked at and listened to with love.

Tinnitus also seems to contain many of the satellite fears we hold already, some of them being:

Claustrophobia: 'I am locked in my own head with this noise. None of my usual escape routes seem to work. I cannot read or talk with others or watch a movie. I cannot get away from this relentless sound…'

Isolation: 'No one understands what I am suffering. I cannot seem to find the words to communicate what I am going through. I am alone. I feel so alone…'

Hopelessness: 'Nothing seems to make it any more bearable. What will I do if it gets worse? How will I cope? I cannot live the rest of my life like this…'

Pain

Tinnitus seems to be a first cousin to pain, 'the ultimate symptom of something else', and the greatest fear of many people. Even death, when one is in pain, seems preferable to suffering.

In the sense that tinnitus may have manifested for any number of deep-seated fears, it is an ideal tool to discover precisely those things you do not want in order to refine precisely what you do indeed desire. This is where you can bring to bear upon your self-guided tour your full abilities as a creator.

This is where you can feel a sense of liberation. Your task is simply to lower your resistance to your well-being. Well-being is here, right now, all around you. All you have to do is allow it in.

Now, how to begin to choose what you want to experience? That's the easy part. It's called **Contrast**, and knowing how to use that contrast consciously is what living well is all about.

7

The Art and Science of Contrast

Whenever a new person enters your life experience and you find them attractive in some way, it's only natural to want to discover more about them; where they come from, what they do for a living, how they think politically, what music, movies or food they like, in order to clarify your reasons for whether or not to spend more time with them.

Looking more deeply, when you meet someone you don't find particularly appealing and feel no interest in knowing more about them, you may realise that you have already, without ever exchanging a word with that person, made a multitude of decisions about them and who they may appear to be.

This is a natural process happening every moment of our lives. Through sight, sound, taste, touch, scent and intuition, we process the information we receive through the filter of past experience and sort it all into many different, and mainly predetermined, categorisations. In our never-ending inner monologue, we often say things like, "Oh, she's a student, that's why she is the way she is." Or, "He's German," or "She's gay," or "He's old…" or, "They're rich; they smell bad; they have a horrible laugh…" and so on.

The same thing happens with every *thing* we observe as well.

In our ongoing love affair with Absolute Truth, we make our categories of preferences very strong and rigid. We feel this process may actually define who we are, so constantly reinforcing these categories is necessary in order to see ourselves as strong individuals. In order to add even more conviction, we also attach the labels "Good" or "Bad" to the category boxes. This ratchets our feelings up a notch, adding the impetus of emotion to the perception of strength. Strawberries are "bad" because the last time you ate them they gave you hives. "Water" is good because it has no calories.

Moving along the scale from fruit and beverages, murderers are "bad" because, well, they kill people. But soldiers are "good" because they kill people for what might seem a valid reason. People who paint pictures of children with no clothes could be "bad," but painted naked infants with wings on the Sistine Chapel ceiling are "good." You can perhaps begin to see how complicated it can get, all this sorting and boxing. Assigning good and bad labels also appears to simplify this massive amount of sensory input.

Returning to our historic need to create our Rock of Absolute Truth, we **up** the intensity of our emotions towards what we decide is good or bad. In order to avoid clinging to our rocks all alone, we also tend to impose our standards of good and bad on others. This is the way that laws are made. This, for the most part, is the way our children are raised. This, for lack of any better way, is how Good Ideas become carved in stone.

Stepping back for a moment, take another look at what might be driving us:

The fear of making a wrong decision; thus the constant reinforcement of categories through heightened emotions labelled 'good' and 'bad.'

The fear of being alone in those decisions; characterised by our desire to impose, either by force or seduction, personally chosen standards upon others.

The fear of being hurt. Strawberries hurt us once. They could hurt us again. Therefore, strawberries are bad. Let's make a law against strawberries. Or not…

Sometimes it gets very tiring. It takes a lot of energy to make and keep our boxes strong. If we feel they define us as humans, though, we will fight to our deaths to maintain them. This leads us to yet another fear-

If we change our beliefs, we might cease to exist.

In one way, that's true. When we change beliefs, the person

we were no longer exists. Put a gentler way, we will simply…change.

If you have to choose an absolute, try this one: The only absolute is change. Try it on for size for a moment. Just a moment. Take it and play with it in your mind and then see how it makes you feel. You can always paddle back to your rock, but let go for just a moment or two and float with it:

The only absolute is change.

An even gentler concept you might play with is this: "It's only fashion." Everything you've ever read or observed or been told is only in fashion right now. Tomorrow it will be different. Why not, really? Our clothes are different, sometimes every month. Think of beliefs as clothes you put on and wear for a while. This will put a whole new light on the phrase "Clothes make the man." If you know anything at all about history you can probably come up with a dozen different examples of how a thing is allowed and even encouraged in one generation, whilst actively prohibited as shameful behaviour in the next. It used to be fashionable to think the sun rotated around a flat earth, or even that the sun was a fiery chariot driven by a god.

Try another one. Instead of 'good' and 'bad,' think of it as contrast. Instead of the often violent emotions attached to good and bad, try loosening the rigidity of your boxes with the terms 'preferred,' or 'not preferred.' This simple re-labelling can afford you the clarity of a more distant perspective, expanding your view a bit and freeing you that much more to be open to change. Don't worry that you may become cold and emotionless, that is not what this is about. When the time comes to apply passion to your creations, you will have that much more to give when you are no longer spending it on hating things in the "bad" category.

Contrast simply exists as a way to select what you desire. The trick to manifesting your desires depends upon where you choose to place your attention and thereby invest your energy. The pain you feel is resistance to the very contrast that exists simply as a means to select what you prefer.

There is nothing either good or bad, but thinking makes it so.
—William Shakespeare.

Just had to throw that quote in. I really like that quote.

During the first few months of my Tinnitus experience I had a lot of time to think. I certainly wasn't socialising, or reading or watching television – two activities only filled my days – searching for information about Tinnitus on the Internet, and thinking while I lay awake at night.

What came to me most clearly throughout this experience was that I had a lot of fearful beliefs in my personal universe, but in total they were all variations on these three:

1. I am not worthy of love.
2. Someone or something is going to hurt me and I will have no power over it.
3. Someday I will die and cease to exist.

I gradually began to realise that, in a way, I had always loved these beliefs. I thought they made me what I am. I depended on them. I identified with them so strongly that I was haunted by the thought that I might cease to exist if they were gone, so I hung on. The cost? Joy. Freedom. Health. It was a pretty steep price to pay for hanging on to what I thought was the essential **me**.

I poured an enormous amount of energy into maintaining a boundary between **Me** and Everything Else. I was living, breathing, working and interacting in this bubble of beliefs defining how I saw myself. The boundary depended upon the concept of protection, illustrated by what existed either inside or outside my personal belief bubble. So much energy and effort, and stress, went into maintaining what I thought of as "myself." I reacted to any threatened breach of the bubble wall in much the same way an astronaut would to a puncture in a spacecraft, or a sailor to a hole in their boat. My fear was that either the outside would rush in and overwhelm me or that what I defined as Me could leak out.

Over the following year I realised that all of these concepts – whether inside or outside of the bubble – were changeable. They were not facts at all, they were only beliefs and could therefore be altered whenever I made the choice.

And here was a clue I discovered when I found myself needing a Rock of Absolute Truth to cling to: The only Fact I ever needed in my universe was my feelings. Everywhere I went I encountered my feelings. This book you are reading is crammed full of my feelings, but like anything else in your life you can chose to read these words and take or leave what you need according to how it makes you feel.

Most of all, everything is changeable, if not reversible. Everything you are experiencing can simply be an episode you pass through, emerging into restored good health on the other side.

Until I was unwell, I hadn't realised I had spent my entire life feeling good. I had spent my entire life not appreciating how good I felt.

The desire to feel good again became my quest. The method was to feel good first and watch my reality change to match it, rather than wearing myself out trying to change reality first in order to feel good. Being versus Doing. You've probably heard it before... the seek-ye-first-the-Kingdom-of-God-and-all-these things-shall-be-added-unto-you sort of thing. And here's a clue; "The Kingdom of God is within you." A really great guy with a really good idea about how the world could work said that.

Tinnitus focused me in the Now Moment, and made me aware of what I truly desired more strongly and more insistently than any experience that I can recall.

So if you are sparing whatever attention span you have available to read these words I have written and find yourself hating the way you feel, sick of the sound in your head, alternately crying or raging, you can begin to change it all right now, in this now moment. I found the blessing that experiencing Tinnitus offered me. Instead of spending my energy hating how

I felt, I pivoted to a place where I began to appreciate what was happening. You can do this too. By using Tinnitus, or any physical dis-ease or discomfort you may ever experience, as an opportunity to focus like a laser upon the Now Moment, you can decide and select what it is you do want, rather than on those things you do not want.

The energy that was previously spent on protection from, avoidance of or hatred for the things I did not desire were transformed to a limitless resource of opportunities for joy by simply seeing contrast where once I only saw 'good' and 'bad.'

The sea of uncertainty will become the ocean of choice and it will then become possible to manifest what you desire with grace and ease and delight.

Are You an Observer of what is, or a Visionary of what could be?

The simplest way to begin is to pay attention to the words you use, both aloud and inside your mind when you think about how you are feeling. Instead of saying, "I hate having this, I hate the way I feel..." try saying, "I love feeling good, I love the way I can hear music and the quiet sound of the wind in the leaves" (or "the shower pounding down on my head," whatever serves you best at the time...).

By focusing at this basic level on what you do desire instead of what you don't, you can change the habits of a lifetime. Make time to be alone, preferably lying down with your eyes closed, and notice your emotions at the time. Are you stressed? Worried? Angry? Feel how that *feels*, get to know that feeling inside and out. Notice how your body is reacting to the way you feel. Are you hot or cold? Are you tense? Are your fists clenched? Does your hair feel like it's standing on end? Really get into the feeling, analyse it, quantify it into a list of physical attributes. When you are certain you know everything you can about the physical symptoms accompanying your present emotion, begin to relax. Don't force yourself to relax, it won't work. Recall every cheesy movie you've ever seen where a hypnotist was telling their subject that their limbs were getting heavy, their eyelids were closing, they were getting sleepy, and so on. Do this now. Sink down into whatever you are lying on. Slow your breathing, concentrating on regular, deep breaths from the diaphragm.

Now, gently, gently…imagine…how you will feel when you are well and whole. Feel how it feels when you glide through your day with ease. Make this scene so real that you could actually be living it. You have permission not only to daydream, but to come as close as you can to virtual reality when you do this. Note the emotions attendant upon what you are imagining. Even better, recall a time in your past when you may have thought, "This is a perfect moment." It may have been when you saw an awe-inspiring sunset in a place you had always longed to be. Or when you kissed that person you had always wanted to kiss and they returned the embrace with a love that seemed to shimmer. Or when you made a perfect score on a test you weren't certain you would do well on. *You have at least one hundred good moments like that in your life, I guarantee it.* Reach into the vast library of your own past experiences and select one of your really good moments. Now feel how you feel. Hold on to that feeling and note how your body is responding. How do you feel? How do you feel? Does it feel like relief? Relief is good, ride that feeling. Develop and expand it by adding colour and texture and detail to your vision of how joy makes you feel.

"Well," you may be saying right about now, "Those good things I am thinking about aren't real, they're just my imagination…"

Of course it's just your imagination. It's also just your imagination when you worry, or fret, when you think about who or what makes you angry and which cutting comment you wish you'd said in response. What's real is how your body responds when you grieve or when you feel guilt, when you are anxious or afraid. Your body becomes tense, develops a headache, gets sick, develops cancer…and you suffer. All because of your imagination. You can now use the power of your imagination to travel the other direction, to make your body glow with health.

It's your choice. It always has been. It always will be. Every single now moment of your life.

And you don't just stop at your physical body. Whether you realise it or not right now, you have used your imagination – through the power of your emotions – to manifest every experience you have ever had. It's just that you may never have made the conscious connection. You may have called it coincidence or synchronicity or hubris, or a score of other terms designed by humans in an attempt to deny the power available to them at all times. You deny it either through fear of the power or from cultural conditioning handed down from people you've allowed to manipulate you for their gain.

Regarding the tendency to deny personal power, it has been a source of continual amazement to me that people seem to readily accept that they can make themselves ill.

People will eagerly say, "Well, I smoked so I got cancer." They may say, "I worried so I got an ulcer...I fretted about everything so I had a stroke...I ate a lot of butter and had a heart attack..." Yet, people, by and large, are reluctant to take credit for making themselves well...they grant that power to others. "The doctor made me well...My prayer group made me well...God made me well..." Hardly ever do you hear anyone say, "I healed myself."

Now all that can change. All you have to do is make the choice and trust the power of your feelings and your ability to envision your desires.

I know I cannot simply say these words and expect you to embrace them. I can only encourage you to discover this gift for yourself and then it will become your truth.

8

Hammer vs Fist

All Tools are Valid, only Some are more Efficient

The only Fact is your Feelings.

Affirmations are like the Swatch Watches of the New Age movement. Everybody's got at least three and most of them just stop working after a while.

Most people, when they obtain or create an affirmation, a really good one that creates a *frisson* of excitement and a feeling of emotional identity, they'll take it for a test drive. They'll meditate with it and tape a printout of it to their bathroom mirror. They'll chant it repeatedly like a Tibetan Buddhist. It may lift them up for a while, then it seems to simply run out of steam. If this has been your experience, you might take a look at how the affirmation is worded. At the most basic level, does it say what you do desire or what you don't desire to happen? Does it say, for example, 'I never get sick,' or does it say, 'I am always healthy'? Does it give you room to re-design your desire?

If you look closely, there's a crucial difference between the two; the phrase 'I never get sick,' contains two words that could send up a red warning signal to your body, the concept of 'never' and the word 'sick.' Same thing with every other desire you may hold in your deepest heart. Take a close look at how you word your desires.

'I don't want to be poor' or 'I would like to have money in free-flowing abundance.'

'I hate being alone' or 'It would be wonderful to see myself lovingly reflected in the eyes of another person.'

The main thing to realise is how your affirmations make you feel. Do they support a sense of what you are lacking or affirm what makes you feel good?

A great deal of emphasis has been placed upon making decisions with your head instead of your heart. It may have been drilled into you all your life that you must face reality, stop day-daydreaming, get it together and use your brain instead of making decisions based on what your feelings . The people and institutions who have taught you this have it backwards when they tell you to think first and feel second. In most cases it is to their advantage to denigrate or eliminate one of the two main resources you are blessed with: how you feel.

In order to create with full awareness those experiences you desire, consistently and with joy, it is necessary to engage both your mind and your feelings, fully and without reservation.

Your brain is a tool best used to sort and select what you truly prefer to experience. Being aware of your feelings, and more to the point, utilising the power of your wonderful brain to *consciously choose* how you feel is how you manifest whatever you desire.

How much time do you spend worrying about being ill? Or physically harmed or destitute and homeless or alone or unloved or embarrassed?

Let's say you don't like peanut butter cookies. Do you spend time worrying that someday, somewhere you will be faced with a peanut butter cookie? Do you develop phobias about peanut butter cookies? Do you invent elaborate scenarios in your mind about how you will react if someday you should go down to your kitchen, open your cookie jar and find a peanut butter cookie in there? No? Then why spend time worrying about anything at all? Everything you ever experience in your life is the result of simple choices you have made between what you prefer to have or not have and, most importantly, **the intensity of feeling motivating those choices.**

"But what about war?" you might be saying about now, "Or disease? Or serial killers or corruption in the marketplace, those are bad things, really bad things that could happen to me anytime. What's all this got to do with what sort of cookie I prefer?"

The difference is the intensity of your feelings and where you choose to focus your attention. You might feel very strongly about disease and place it in the box you label *Very Bad Things That Must Be Avoided At All Costs.* You have less negative emotional attachment to peanut butter cookies, so you place that item in the *Cookies I'd Rather Not Eat Because I like Other Cookies Better* box.

The trouble comes with the intensity of feeling invested in the things that are 'Bad, Very Bad'.

I'm going to tell you the secret of the Universe now. Just like that. I am going to tell you why things are the way they are.

I realise I probably should have placed this in its own category, perhaps in a special chapter entitled 'This Is The Reason Everything Is The Way It Is in Your Life,' including elaborate charts and diagrams, or footnotes, or a bibliography, or at the very least an impressive gothic font. Instead, I am just sliding it in here with little-to-no fanfare. Nevertheless, that's the way really profound things often appear in life, little clues popping up just at the corner of your eyesight just as you were about to glance away. These clues are often subliminal, nearly subtext, these hints that have been there all along, tapping you on the shoulder or... ringing in your ear...

Here it is. Are you ready?

The secret to the way that your life, the universe and everything works is this:

Everything, *everything* is all about Law of Attraction.

The Law of Attraction states that like is drawn to like. There is no 'Law of Get it Away From Me,' there is only the Law of Attraction.

What does this mean? It means that if you are constantly concerned with the bad things that might happen, if you are afraid that if you relax your vigilance even for an instant some catastrophe will take place, then *you will draw those experiences to you through the attention and focus you give them by avoiding and dreading and continually thinking about the possibility that they might occur.* The universe doesn't know bad from good, it only knows vibrations of energy. How you vibrate, through the feelings you choose and your attention to those feelings, is what creates the thing you define as your reality.

Everything you have ever experienced in this life, you have created from your feelings *first*, whether or not you were aware of it at the time. That's why I'm suggesting it might be preferable to create consciously. You are creating everything anyway, all the time. We had the victim chat earlier in the book, yes? And you've decided it's time to open your heart and mind to a new possibility, the possibility that there are no victims, only creators.

So, here you are, reading these words, feeling like you might be beginning to get it, wondering if it could be true and possibly feeling the same tingling excitement you experience just before you open a treasure chest or unwrap a gift from someone you love and...

It's true. You create everything that happens to you. Whether or not you create it consciously can now be your choice.

Doing a You-Turn

A person dear to you may have died in a car accident and this affected you profoundly for ever after. At some point you may decide to make a conscious decision that the past accident belonged to that person's reality and does not necessarily have to be a part of your experience as well. You make the conscious decision to focus your attention upon feelings of security, peace and joy. You will then no longer be 'destined' to be in a car accident. There is no fear anymore either in your heart or in your mind. On the day an accident happens it will now happen without you. You won't be there. You will, instead, be strutting along, seeing the world as a beautiful place filled with opportunities for joy and instead of being in the car accident you were vibrating towards before, events have re-aligned so that you take the bus instead of riding in that accident-bound car. Or the person who offered to pick you up at the airport before crashing into another car is running late and you decide to take a cab instead. A hundred million bazillion things will be different than they would have been if you were grooving the 'car accident' vibe. And it all happens easily, effortlessly and elegantly, without pain or suffering or striving to make it happen. All purely from the power of your ability to focus upon what you desire instead of what you try to avoid.

For every 'accident' you have ever experienced, there are countless near or complete misses of accidents that you will never know about because you weren't vibrating with fear about that particular topic. Been attacked by any peanut butter cookies lately? No? Just asking. Play with that thought anyway. It won't cost anything and might just notch up your appreciation levels for how good life really is. You walk, drive, run, breathe, sleep, eat, laugh, bathe, shop, travel and drink pure, clean water all day, everyday and nothing terrible happens, right? That's good, right? Of course it's good...if it feels good to think it. And the more you think it and feel it, the more good experiences will take place in your life. The more things will turn around into experiences of joy.

You might be asking yourself right about now how I could possibly know all this is true. How do I know it's real? What makes me so special?

*How do I know **you**, Elspeth Fahey, aren't a mentally deranged person full of bullshit and trying to make a buck out of my gullibility?*

Well, I suppose the simple answer is, you don't.

All you ever know is how it makes you feel.

If what I have written makes you feel good, then it's right for you. If it makes you feel bad, then I expect you would have stopped reading by now.

Getting back to vibrating and attracting and consciously choosing how you feel and appreciating all the good there is to being alive in this now moment, you might take a look at the quantum mechanical view of life, the universe and everything in relation to the individual.

Oh good, science.

I love science. I fall asleep to science programmes on BBC2 Open University nearly every night. Here we go:

Time and space and the events that occur in relation to the span of both are fluid, they change moment to moment and each now moment is a new opportunity to make a new choice. The briefest glance at quantum theory will validate this view. The relatively recent discovery that the act of observation, as influenced by the vibratory rate of the individual observer, makes a quantifiable difference on the outcome of any given experiment was a real stunner when it was announced to the world-wide scientific community. Stated in simpler terms, what you expect to see, you see. No scientist goes into observation mode completely free of some anticipated outcome, thereby influencing the result of any given experiment.

Can that be true? Are we really that powerful? Could everything that happens to our bodies and our life experience be…a habit of thought? Could it be that simple?

And now, for my next science trick, I want to talk about probabilities. In a quantum mechanical world, no one can predict where a particle will be with 100% certainty. They can only speak in terms of probabilities. For example, they can say that an atom will be at some location with a 99% probability, but there will be a 1% probability it will be somewhere else – in fact, there will be a small but finite probability that it will be found across the Universe. Where science has fallen to its knees and howled at the moon for so many centuries is due to the belief that there is a separation between the subatomic and the macroscopic world. There is no difference at all. As above, so below, it is all connected. The larger picture, the smallest particle. All is one.

Every island is a mountaintop. Beneath the ocean of consciousness we are all connected. The islands of what we perceive as separate existence are an illusion born of desire to experience ourselves as individual. The experience of being an individual is where – in this now moment – we hold the power of conscious creation.

The only thing holding us back from accomplishing anything we desire is the belief that we are powerless and the fear that if we believe in miracles we will be disappointed.

Before every manifestation into 'reality' is the feeling and the inspiration. Motivating them both is the pure desire of an individual soul.

Look around you, do you see the building you are in? Before it was bricks or walls or a roof, before it was plumbing and electricity, it was an idea in someone's head inspired by a desire in their heart. The same goes for everything around you. First it was the feeling of desire, then an inspiration, then a reality.

A really super thing just happened to me. I went into the kitchen to make a cup of tea. Redbush tea. In South Africa, the only place on earth where redbush tea feels like growing right now, it's called Rooibos tea. It's great. It's a pretty colour and it tastes good and it's eleven times higher in antioxidants than green tea and you can drink it with milk just like regular tea except that it doesn't have any caffeine, which is nice in the evening. All in all, it's just about every good thing a tea ought to be and often isn't.

Anyway, here in the UK there is this neat little car you can buy, very tiny, very cute and it's called the Smart Car. On this particular box of redbush tea I just noticed an advertisement for a contest in which you could win the new model of Smart Car, the *Smart Passion*. I just read this and rushed back in to tell you all about it.

This is what I have been banging on about while I typed this chapter... Smart Passion... the ability to consciously engage both your mind and your feelings to create the alchemy of manifestation of desire. Smart Passion. Anyway, for the price of a box of tea I thought it was a pretty affordable epiphany.

Life can be full of moments like that when you open all three eyes.

9

You Are Never Finished Creating

It takes a selfish person to want to feel good. Feeling good should become your quest. You cannot create any other person's reality, your power lies in the creation of your own life experience, always, in this now moment. Conversely, to depend on any other person to supply and maintain your happiness is not only complicated and cumbersome but ultimately disappointing.

Nearly everyone who's ever played a game feels the desire to test the parameters. Computer games are a great metaphor for your life experience, particularly the ones where you can design your character before you begin play. You assign this character certain attributes and abilities and then turn them loose; as you choose the attributes that define your character you may ask yourself what would happen if you're the bad guy? How would it feel if you cheated? What would it be like to shoot everything in sight, to be killed, to abort the game? So we try all those things. We test and reconfigure and try again in order to see how it feels because...

Feelings make us alive, and how we feel about anything is a living, fluid choice in every moment.

Everyone plays the game of life, though only the people who admit they are playing will ever win their dearest desires. Your life is a game and you are writing (and re-writing) the rules every moment. You are playing a game where the only competition is yourself. Sort of lightens things up a bit, doesn't it? Well it should. It's a game. You cannot get it wrong and you will never really lose because there is no death and desire never ends.

Desire

The family in which I grew up repeatedly stressed two things. One was, "Count your blessings" and the other was the question "Aren't you ever satisfied?"

Looking back at that time from the lofty heights of "adulthood" I would have to answer "OK" to the first and "Uh...no, I'm not satisfied..." to the second. No, I'm not satisfied, not in a final never-need-to-change-another-thing sort of way.

Looking at the first statement, "Count your blessings," the inference was "Be grateful for what you've got 'cause think how bad you'd feel if you didn't have it anymore." Since my childhood I have come to realise that counting my blessings can open the way to appreciation. Appreciation is one of the main motivators to quickly pivot from a place of seeing the bad, the dangerous and the threatening to a place of seeing more that is good and wonderful in my life. Appreciation turns my focus from a place of lack to a vista of abundance. I am grateful for this lesson. It was a jewel in a wrapping of common canvas.

The other concept, "Aren't you ever satisfied?" has since become transformed into the realisation of the precious gift of desire. Desire is good. Desire turns on our inner light. Desire and the deliciousness of anticipation is the yummy good feeling we all want again and again. It is the eternal Christmas Eve before the gifts are opened.

When desire is born from a place of lack, nurtured in a place of the persistent feeling that *if you only had this thing you desired, then you could be happy*, it can leave most people with a sense of letdown (and/or maxed-out credit cards) once that desire is fulfilled. They find they are not any happier than they were before and avidly seek the next 'thing' they hope might fill the void they feel inside.

Through the power of appreciation, you can pivot from any seemingly negative experience to a place of joy. From this place of joy you can give birth to the desire to experience something else wonderful. When you desire from a place of joy you not only enjoy the manifestation of your desire, *you enjoy the journey of anticipation*. When the manifestation arrives, this creates a launching pad of joy for the next desire to be manifested. And the next. And the next. Constantly creating, preferring, desiring, sifting the contrast and fine-tuning the next fun experience.

Feelings make us alive. Feeling joy *before the manifestation* makes being alive everything it is supposed to be in our greatest, grandest dreams.

Responsibility and Culpability

One of the most popular life games, as introduced earlier, is Victim. It's a best-seller and most of us have become so good at it that we've forgotten it's a game. Sometimes we've been playing it so long we've forgotten other games even exist. There is something seductive about the Victim Game. It's expected. It's ingrained. It's currently fashionable. It feels familiar and we know the rules.

Would you like some new rules? Here is a starter set directly from my life experience:

Culpability is blame.

Responsibility is self-love.

Culpability is guilt.

Responsibility is the conscious self-recognition of personal power.

Victims play with culpability. Creators deal in responsibility.

When people are told "You should take responsibility..." they most often hear "Accept punishment for fill-in-the-blank." As a result, most people spend so much time and energy running from the former (culpability) that they rarely stop and embrace the latter (responsibility). Most people live much of their lives feeling like either a victim of something or a perpetrator of something else.

Don't confuse culpability and responsibility. They are two entirely separate things.

In the source code of social programming depended upon by many people to interpret their reality, whenever some threat to existence presents itself, their first instinct is to find someone to blame. This usually takes the form of justifying why they are right, sometimes reasonably, sometimes with violence, in an attempt to garner support for their view. This search for social approbation, and ultimately, recompense for perceived injury, can escalate from a simple campaign or debate or publicity for your cause all the way to a formal lawsuit tried in a court of law.

When groups of people feel threatened, offended or injured, the source code tells them they need to find someone to blame *and make them pay for what they've done.*

In an effort to codify correct modes of behaviour in society, laws are enacted and, more or less, enforced in every community.

As a conscious creator, as a thriver, what is your personal responsibility to the laws enacted by a government, community, tribe, club or family? Whatever you feel your responsibility should be. Whatever feels good, and I mean *good, right, and joyous for you* deep inside your being. This precludes doing what you are compelled to do by anger, or a need to rebel against what you see as power held over you, or in retaliation against what you perceive your parents or your spouse or your president or your boss or your priest have done to you. That stuff doesn't feel good, so why would you be inspired to act from it?

Why settle for recompense when you can have joy? Joy is born from loving yourself. Recompense is sought when you feel powerless.

If everyone loved themselves and lived lives of joy, there would be no need for laws. People who require a strong system of laws do not, as a rule, feel safe from their own inner urgings, needs or desires and require outside constructs to repress those desires.

It is interesting to observe that as more laws are enacted, more prisons seem to be built. It is often difficult to find one person who has never broken some law, sometime, somewhere. It is clear that people are going to do what people are going to do and all the laws in the world aren't going to make those desires go away.

No one can force change or conformity upon anyone else. If this were truly realised, most of the problems of this world would cease to exist and all laws and the need to enforce them would no longer be necessary.

No one is culpable. Everyone is responsible. That the two are so often used interchangeably is evidence of old source code programming which you can consciously choose to change.

And now, just a little bit more science before I stop and go hug a tree.

"It will happen. You will bask in well-being for longer and longer periods like I have. And all the cells of your body will respond to match your feeling."

This is a statement that generally makes left-brain, analytical thinkers curl their toes and turn aside in mild distaste at best and strong disdain at worst. I understand.

Since the dark ages, and the dawning of the Age of Reason, humans have had a long-term love affair with the Cartesian and Newtonian views of reality. Keeping that in mind, I now present, for your edification and entertainment, more cool science stuff that people with actual degrees agree on:

Science has proved that the cells of the pancreas shed and regenerate 100% every 24 hours...every single day we have an entirely new pancreas. The stomach lining is completely regenerated every four days and the liver every six weeks.

With this scientifically validated evidence of perpetual regeneration and opportunity for change, how did I make this wonderful knowledge serve my desire for the silencing of tinnitus?

I simply changed my habit of thought about tinnitus being permanent, about hair cells not being able to regenerate, about everything that had to do with the nature of change and healing, I learned to expect it to happen without fear of disappointment or failure, I imagined with my entire being how good health feels and my cells followed suit to match this new vibration.

So I will say it again.

"It will happen. You will bask in well-being for longer and longer

periods like I have. And all the cells of your body will respond to match your feeling."

Self-love will change your world, and *Your World* is all you ever need be concerned with

Being loved is a choice you make for yourself. It cannot be bought or sold or bargained for. It must be given to yourself, from yourself before you are ready to receive it from another.

Regarding many relationships, one of the reasons people often say, "Opposites attract..." is that most people look to another person to supply what they feel they lack. An introverted person may have a vivacious or gregarious partner or a person looking for financial security may choose a partner richer than they are.

Often it's more complex than this. (Isn't everything suddenly more complex once you grant a person access to previously unexplored levels of intimacy?) Some people seek in a partner a way to resolve issues in their past, particularly any unhappy associations with their parents. To this end, an individual may set their partner up as either their parental ideal or as an arbiter of relationship protocol and embark upon a campaign to acquire and keep their approval.

As you know, this often, if not always, ends in tears – or at the very least, disillusionment. Whenever you set another person on a pedestal, you set yourself up in a position of needing their approval, and need is the purest form of slavery there is. In any situation you may encounter in the relationship, the instant you need the other person to say the words **I love you** or **I want you** or **You're beautiful** or **I'm sorry**, then you have handed them the power to decide whether or not you can be happy.

If you don't feel loved or desirable first, inside yourself, then the other person can say these things to you a million and twelve times and you'll never be able to believe it or really enjoy hearing it, because – deep inside – you suspect it isn't true.

Some people love this slavery game, though. *Really* love it. For many it approaches or surpasses the pleasure of the sexual act. An entire subculture has been built and is maintained by and for people to play out their dominant/submissive desires.

If you are not one of these people, if you haven't elevated this desire to an art form that brings you joy, you might look carefully and see if you are continually placing partner after partner on a pedestal and subsequently attacking the base of this pedestal with a sledgehammer. If you are, it could be time to explore what it is you think you may lack and hope that some other person can supply.

When you discover that any perceived lack is only a belief and that your birthright is the ability to create everything you desire, you will then attract people who will enhance your life, rather than appear to supplement what you fear you lack. You will manifest a relationship free to become that which serves both of you best in terms of joy, as well as creating an adventure of personal and mutual discovery.

Being loved is a choice you make for yourself. It cannot be bought or sold or bargained for. It must be given to yourself, from yourself before you are ready to receive it from another.

If you firmly believe you are unable to change your past then you can always change your *feelings* about the past.

I am a profoundly lazy person so I have designed exercises you can do lying down very still with your eyes shut, because if it can be imagined with positive passion – *smart passion* – then it will most certainly be manifested as reality in your own life. There's no need whatsoever to ever break a sweat over anything again. Unless you are still attached to the old idea that a thing not earned is a thing not worth having… you can change it now.

non-exercise 1

letting it go

Gently stop guiding or monitoring what you are thinking and instead, pay attention to how your body reacts to what you are thinking. Lie down in a comfortable place and allow your thoughts to run the way they will. Be aware of what your body is doing…is your jaw clenched? Does your foot twitch? Can you feel tension in your lower back? Consciously relax these places, letting your body sink and open. Pay attention to your breathing, is it shallow and quick? Is it full, rolling breaths? Give yourself permission to daydream, let your mind wander, occasionally checking in mentally on what your body is doing. Do your fantasies begin happily enough, then transform into can-nots, should-nots or fear? What is your body doing now? Relax and begin again, aware at every moment where you hold tension and resistance. Doing this regularly in a safe environment like your bed will help you be aware of your stress level when you go out into the world. Soon it will become first nature to you to relax in whatever situation you might find yourself in.

non-exercise 2

begin noticing those little "coincidences"

Like the tea I described earlier with the car advertisement, you will begin to notice seeming coincidences in your life directly relating to your inner work. These are clues and signs that you are on the right track. Parking spaces will appear when you need them, you will arrive at appointments precisely on time, the person you really desire to speak with will ring on the phone and, what's more, you will "know" it's them as you pick it up to answer.

The apparent opposite of good coincidences are true as well. Have you ever noticed how a bad day begins and often keeps getting worse? You can choose in each moment to take notice of this trend and turn it all around by changing your focus to the positives you desire. Don't spend any more time beating yourself up for getting it wrong, it is simply part of the contrast that is your most valuable tool to refine precisely what you do desire to experience.

non-exercise 3

accentuate the positive

You might have to open your eyes and actually sit up to do this, but it's not all that strenuous so give it a go. Write on a piece of paper all the positive things you can think of about, say, a person you have had a difficult time with. Think of every good thing you can come up with about them and write it down. Begin noticing those good points at every opportunity. As this becomes more and more natural to you, one of two amazing things will happen, either that person will seemingly vibrate right out of your life or they will **appear to change** right before your eyes. If they have scampered, it then becomes entirely up to you whether or not they come back into your life. If you return to your previous vibration you might find they have clattered right back in and you are back where you started, in an unhappy and unsatisfactory relationship. Don't get caught up in trying to make them happy so you can be happy because it will never work, you can only make yourself happy and the other person either matches that vibration or they beat feet right out of your life. Happens every time, I guarantee it. This also works with cars, pets, weather, health, career, anything you experience in your life. Make a list of positives and your world will change to suit your most passionate desire for joy.

non-exercise 4

virtual reality

This is where the rubber meets the metaphysical road.

We get so caught up in **doing,** running around frantically all through our lives trying to **make** things happen when there is a much easier and more elegant road to take. We've been taught to believe that intense visualisation is only daydreaming, the retreat of the terminally lazy no-account.

Hear this, know this: Everything begins with a feeling inspired by a thought. You can make the absolute best and balanced use of both halves of yourself, head and heart, by consciously choosing thoughts that feel better. Your only task is to feel good. Feel good. Feel good.

My favourite teacher has said,

"On your deliberately joyous journey your actions will be inspired, your resources will be abundant and you will know by the way you feel that you are fulfilling your reason for life. Most have this one backwards, therefore most feel little joy in their actions or their possessions. Your loving, Inner Being offers guidance in the form of emotion. Entertain a wanted or unwanted thought and you feel a wanted or unwanted emotion. Choose to change the thought and you've changed the emotion and the creation."

So begin to embrace the concept that your thoughts hold the power to design your universe and devote three minutes to this exercise. For three minutes relax, breathe with an open, relaxed rhythm and immerse yourself in a total mental picture of what you would most desire to have. Do not get caught up in **how to make it happen**, visualise it already accomplished, ride that wave and feel how that feels. Smell it, touch it, taste it, embrace it, roll around and rub it in your hair if you like, but **be the experience** for three minutes. This is the first half of conscious creation, the second half is to allow it in.

And how to allow? Remain positive. Pet your cat, fly a kite, play in the rain, write a list of positives, take a hot bath, it will come to you when you are consistently vibrating the joy that allows more joy in.

Gnothi Seauton

Now... if you really **enjoy** being hard on yourself, you might be more comfortable with the drill sergeant approach. If you feel like you are accomplishing things more efficiently by playing the tough guy then do it constructively by asking those hard questions you spend so much time and effort avoiding...here's a list that might get you started...

With every choice I make, am I trying to distract myself from pain and boredom or am I enhancing my life by choosing what I really desire to experience?

What am I trying not to hear?

How important is it to me to have the approval of other people in order to feel good about myself?

How important is **being right** to me? How important is it to

be seen to be right?

Have I calculated the cost of setting myself up to be admired?

Am I afraid of dying?

How many times have I turned on the television, not because there was something I wished to see, but because I was bored?

When was the last time I really laughed?

How many times have I gone in search of something to eat or drink not because I was hungry or thirsty, but because I was upset?

How many times have I gone out not because I wanted to have fun, but because I hate being alone?

What am I trying to distract myself from thinking or feeling?

On the other hand, isn't it more fun to imagine all the things that are right about your life, *right now*, than to spend any more time focussing on what seems to be "wrong?"

I say, go fly a kite!

Hot Damn, I'm Enlightened! Then Why did I just Stub my Toe?

Sometimes, when you make a major change in your approach to life, it seems to open the floodgates to what you have been holding back all these years. That's all it is, a flood of change and further opportunities to decide from the point of contrast exactly what you do desire. That's step one in creating, that sudden blast of contrast. It's a powerful feeling, it's a load of energy... relax into it.

Step two is turning your attention away from all the things you don't desire and focussing purely and completely on what would bring you joy. Devote those magic few minutes to doing this as described in the VR exercise above.

Step three is simply letting it in...not questioning when it's going to come, or how it's going to come, or why it isn't here yet, but distracting your attention from the lack of what you desire by doing something that brings you pleasure.

Everyone's heard of the couple who tries for years to get pregnant and give birth and this ability seems, through any number of possible reasons, to elude them. Then, when they finally give up trying so hard, and they adopt a child, that is the time when the woman finally conceives. From 'no babies' they have gone to 'two babies' in relatively little time. This often happens because they have turned their attention from **Lack of Child** in their lives to its opposite, and the energy of creation and law of attraction step in and brings more abundance than they may have originally planned.

In creating what you desire, why stop at tinnitus? Why not create a slender, youthful body, a strong heart and muscles and joints...you can have anything. If it can be imagined, felt and allowed, it can be manifested. Bask in the feeling of joyous health in every part of your body, allow it in by focussing on whatever makes you tingle with joy **and all the cells of your being will respond to match that vibration.**

Homo Sapiens to Homo Spiritus, or My Nineteenth Nervous Breakthrough

If you are waiting for the world to be perfect, you will never see perfection again. If you are waiting for no one to be corrupt, you will never trust again. If you are waiting for world peace, you will be waiting forever, for there will always be others who want to play at war. Whether or not you play along is entirely your choice. No one, at any time, ever holds power over you unless you allow it. No one can ever hurt you unless you allow it. There is no death. Life is forever. You cannot get it wrong. You never get it done. Aiming to be perfect? Finished with being a self-creator? You may as well ask yourself when you will be finished looking things up on the Internet! If you want to see God, you don't have to go any further than your mirror. There is always more to discover, to desire, to dream of and create. You are beautifully and perfectly incomplete. You are eternal and you are surrounded at all times by the love you have always desired.

Your only task is to allow in this love and wellbeing by consciously choosing your feelings, by always choosing, above all things, to feel good. **Be selfish enough** to feel good, always.

Time for tea.

All Fool's Day, 2003

Acknowledgements

Many thanks to Dr Ng Keng Teong, Dr Ng Keng Leong, Dr Ng Keng Jin, Dr Bethan Suyin Thomas, Lan Yin Thomas, Michael Quinlan, Jupiter Jones, Catherine Cheron Dirkx, Po Shun Leong, Doris Cain, Gerald Cain, Bill Gilmer, Kim Corbet, Andy Feehan, Charles Dvorsky, Cathy S. Birn and Abraham through Esther and Jerry Hicks.

Printed in the United States
65603LVS00002B/38

9 781905 605033